Multiple Myeloma

The plain English Handbook for Patients and Care Givers

Robert J. Heller

Multiple Myeloma
The Plain English Handbook
for Patients and Care Givers

Second Edition
Copyright 2005
Wollaston Press

ISBN 0-9657005-3-4

Wollaston Press
4013 Coyte Court
Marietta, GA 30062

DEDICATION

For Phyllis and for all the tens of thousands
of families who are compelled to deal with
this insidious disease.

And with deep appreciation for all of the
medical teams who toil ceaselessly to
find the cure. May the day soon come
when Multiple Myeloma is recalled like
Polio or Small Pox.

FORWARD

I am sorry that you are reading this handbook, because it means that somebody you care deeply about has been plunged into the morass called Multiple Myeloma. As somebody who is in the depths of that experience as this is written, I wish you a speedy and easy route to a complete remission.

You will find references in this work to my wonderful wife, Phyllis. You'll find Phyllis and me on the back cover. This is a handbook written from real life experiences. It's the net sum of our learning to the date of publication or revision.

When we first learned that she was diagnosed with Stage-3 Multiple Myeloma I hit the bookstores seeking information. I found nothing written in easy to understand English. I hit the internet, and found an over-supply of information in which I almost drowned until I began to sort it all out.

Some of it was written like this passage I found in a hematology site. *"In Section III, Dr. F reviews apoptotic pathways as they relate to MM therapy. Defects in the mitochrondrial intrinsic pathway result from imbalances in expression levels of Bcl-2, Bcl-XL and Mcl-1. Mcl-1 is a candidate target gene for rapid induction of apoptosis by flavoperidol. Antisense oglionucleotides (ASO) lead to the rapid induction of caspace activity and apoptosis, which was potentiated by dexamethasone. Similar clinical trials with Bcl-2 ASO molecules alone and in combination with doxorubicin and dexamethasone or thalidomide showed promising results."*

Now if you can actually understand some of that, you don't need this primer. The rest of us mere mortals find the foregoing a bit daunting, and hence the need for some plain talk.

I didn't put a Table of Contents in this book because I want you to go through all of it. And you may find that I repeat a few things which I feel are important, and that's because you may pick up the book and refer to a single section some day and I don't want you to miss the point.

I want to make sure you know that just like the prescription bottles which always seem to have a couple of little yellow warning labels on them (which few ever read) that this handbook comes with two cop-outs. I am not a doctor and this publication is not intended to provide medical instruction or advice. Don't mess around with MM, make sure you have competent care. Also, no printed publication relating to MM could possibly be totally up to date because new advances are being made each month and by the time the ink would dry there would be something missing from any book. So use this as a starting point, not an encyclopedia.

Bob Heller

OUCH

You've just been hit by a bus while crossing a street, or maybe somebody whacked you on the side of your head with a brick. That's about how we felt when we were first told that Phyllis had been diagnosed with something called Multiple Myeloma.

Nobody ever heard of this disease unless he were some kind of cancer specialist or had a family member afflicted with it. It's one of the most rare and insidious forms of cancer and the prognosis is not quite what you wish it would be. But as you fall into that black pit of doubt, uncertainty and fear you soon find there is light at the end of the tunnel and it isn't necessarily that of an incoming freight train.

If you live in a major urban area you will probably find there are medical specialists who are knowledgeable about Multiple Myeloma (MM). There are support groups in many cities and countries. There are several research foundations, and quite a bit of medical information. Unfortunately for we laymen, it is sometimes true that a little knowledge can be a dangerous thing. It can also be a mind-fuddling thing when it is written in medical lingo which isn't really easily understood by the rest of us mere mortals.

When I started to write this book my wife and I were going through a lot of the same stuff you will experience. I am not a physician. I am pretty bright, but as I started to dig into the subject for us, I really yearned for somebody who would try to tell us just what was happening in plain language.

The first clues were a "spiking" in the blood work which was spotted by our primary care physician who referred us to a hematologist-oncologist at a cancer center. We approached that visit with some trepidation, as anything with the "Big C" is something we all want to stay away from. The physical observations, symptoms and blood work were all so right-on with MM that there was no room left for reasonable doubt even though a final diagnosis could not be pronounced until the bone marrow biopsy had been returned. Each of us in the room knew that this alien force called MM had invaded her body, and would have to be counter-attacked with every weapon at our disposal.

The oncologist advised us in that meeting that MM was not curable and of the then accepted 2-year and 5-year survival rates, and that was like being hit again with a sledge hammer. You don't have to be Albert Einstein to figure out that if a survival rate for any number of years is 40%; then 60% of the group are deceased within that time. This can only be equated in impact to being sentenced without benefit of trial or counsel.   So the very first thing you need to know is that any survival rate is an arithmetic mean average which may include those who pass on within a month or two, as well as those who are alive and enjoying life 15 or more years after diagnosis.

It is after the initial shock wears off that we start to dig in to find out just what can be done to prevent further damage, restore prior vitality and retain quality of life.   We quickly learn that no two patients are the same, and the progress of this disease is somewhat unpredictable in relation to treatment.   MM is not like a broken limb that gets set, put in a cast, and heals itself up in time.   It is quite possibly the most enigmatic disease in the world.   It is presumed to account for less than 1% of all cancers, and afflicts about 4 out of every 100,000 persons in the general population.

Is MM related to some environmental cause?   There doesn't seem to be any evidence of that to date.   Phyllis is a stained glass artist and in the course of that avocation she works with lead and zinc; and I was concerned these metals might have some influence. It would appear that MM is totally enigmatic in its origins and not connected to non-ferrous metals, insulating materials, dental fillings, or oil spills. Whether or not nuclear waste is a factor is something we won't really know about for a long time.

We also have to ask if it is genetic in nature. The short answer is, No it is not. Just because a sibling had prostate cancer or breast cancer has little influence upon your chances of later being diagnosed with MM. Conversely, the fact that nobody in your family history has ever had a cancer is no guarantee that you will not become a MM patient.

Your lifestyle has nothing to do with this disease, either. If you are overweight, drink a bit too often, smoke stuff you shouldn't smoke, enjoy boating on closed waters or keep animals none of that is deemed as contributing to the incidence of MM.

The plain truth is that this is an insidious disease, which seemingly strikes at random. Its progress may be slow or extremely rapid. It is serious. It is not curable. And having all that to deal with the next step is to know that many MM patients are survivors of many years beyond the statistical survival rates mentioned before.

The amount of money going into MM research is a lot less than that dedicated to breast cancer, AIDS, or other big time diseases. However, the advances made in the past decade are incredible and the rate at which new ground is being broken in recent years suggests that a far clearer picture of effective treatment may be a possibility in the near future.

What remains true at the time of this writing is that MM is a terrible and frightening journey. It is an attempt to escape from a strange, dark and evil wood at night, while blindfolded, with no road map, where no roads or trails are marked, and where no signs are placed to advise how far you have progressed or have yet to travel. It is frightening, confusing, and can fill one with so many different emotions.

And that is about the point where we declare we shall not yield. We shall learn. We shall fight. We shall prevail to the best of our abilities. And in that fight, Phyllis and I sincerely hope that this book will be of some help and support to you on this terrible journey.

You will find several Appendices at the back of the book that contain contact information and reproducible forms which you will find of use. If you are the patient, know that there are sincere helping hands and hearts out there who want to help you survive this onslaught. If you are the care giver, know that you and your loved one are not alone. The journey may not be as physically demanding for you as for your loved one, but is bound to be emotionally draining and that you, too, will find many who wish to help you both through this terrible journey.

So let us start out. . . .

THIS CAN'T BE
HAPPENING TO ME

This can't be happening to me.   How can the doctors really know?   There must be some other problems that would manifest themselves with similar symptoms.   And why didn't that other doctor find this when he saw me some months ago?

All very common initial reactions and very common questions.   There are objective tests such as images of the bones, and detailed blood and urine analyses that are used to confirm the diagnosis of MM.   There are subjective evaluations such as persistent pain, unexplained fractures, loss of height, recurrent infections and chronic fatigue which may signal MM.   These may not be definitive in and of themselves, but when accompanied by the more objective tests you add them all together and the conclusion becomes inescapable.   If you have any doubts, by all means you have the right, if not the obligation to yourself, to obtain a second opinion.   Any doctor should be willing to give you the images, reports, his notes and other materials to be reviewed by another physician.

Myeloma is usually defined as a cancer of the blood. More specifically it is a cancer which affects the plasma cells and it is the plasma cells in which antibodies mature which help to keep us healthy and thwart many diseases. It is the immunoglobulins produced by these plasma cells which fight infection and illness. There are thousands of different types of plasma cells in your body as each one is formed to fight off a specific foreign substance. When the development of these plasma cells goes awry we have myeloma which is the production of malignant plasma cells. This is an over-simplification, as there are more than one type of cell which are derived from a stem cell, and within these cells there are different types of immunoglobulins which develop. You may hear your doctor referring to a kappa or lambda light or heavy chain which refers to the actual internal structure of the cell itself.

One type of stem cell is called a B cell. It is thought this cell is the one which permits the malignant myeloma cells to be formed. When the system which produces the B cells goes haywire, it starts to produce some damaged, or malformed plasma cells which then start to multiply unchecked and overpopulate their normal living space. The act of over producing is the malignancy. They are now producing a mess of immunoglobulins which the

15

body doesn't need. And here is where the trouble really starts.

Plasma cells normally reside in your bone marrow which is the soft stuff found deep within your bones. Myeloma cells are distinguished from healthy cells in that they have an adhesion molecule which permits them to grow in bone marrow and attack your bones. Normally the plasma cells make up only about 5% of the cells in your bone marrow. But when MM is present it may run well over 50%.

The actual growth scenario is fairly complex and not particularly important to a patient. Basically the diseased cells make themselves at home and feed off cells in the bone marrow called stromal cells. As the myeloma cells multiply they need more blood to foster their growth and they start to create more blood vessels to increase the supply lines and now you have a tumor growing.

As the population of myeloma cells increases it starts to invade the hard part of the bone and they also invade any small cavities in the skeletal structure. These tumors, or lesions, are the essence of MM. A single tumor is referred to as plasmacytoma, while MM refers to the disease being found in multiple sites within the body.

MM is thought to start with a single bad cell which starts to reproduce unchecked. Each such bad cell that is formed is an exact clone of the one from which it arose and will produce the same unneeded immunoglobulin. The immunoglobulin protein is usually referred to as monoclonal, and may be also referred to by the type of immunoglobulin and light chain which it is found to be producing.

Dr. Morie Gertz of the Mayo Clinic likens MM to a garden which is overgrown by weeds and in his depiction the weeds start to take over the ground previously occupied by the good plants. As the weeds will grow unchecked, they finally suck up all the nutrients and force the good plants into second place. As they then continue their growth unchecked, they will wind up invading the barriers of the garden, be they wood or other materials. We've all seen weeds growing right through cement sidewalks so we can relate to how invasive they can become.

I think of MM more as a termite invasion. The termites find your home. They start to move in and as they get more comfortable they start eating up the home in which they find themselves. Myeloma cells do much the same as they invade the bone marrow and then the bones and break down the hardest bones as they expand their operations.

And, like dealing with termites, we usually find out after some initial damage has been observed and we call in the exterminators and then the repair crews. The analogy continues as we are diagnosed with MM, we then move first to stop any further destruction, then to kill off the invaders, and finally to rebuild the body.

Myeloma is fairly obscure attacking about 15,000 people a year in the USA. And that may be one reason why you never heard of MM until it invaded your home. 250 cases a week isn't a headline grabber compared to breast cancer or multiple sclerosis. It usually attacks people over the age of 50, hits men more than women, and blacks more than whites.

The early stage symptoms of MM are elusive. Patients often will experience lower back or other bone pain, become anemic and fatigued, or just keep getting a string of infections. As a result, they get treated for unspecified pain, get put on diet programs, and fed plenty of infection fighting medicines. In the meantime the termites are ignoring these efforts and they continue with their work.

There are various diagnostic tests which are used to confirm the presence of MM in a patient. The first you will encounter is a Complete Blood Count (CBC) and you will have many of these done in the course of your treatment. See the form at the back of this book which you can use to keep a record of these counts.

The CBC measures various aspects of your blood including, but not limited to, red blood cells, white cells, and platelets. In the glossary you will find a brief description of each of the more common aspects of a CBC. Those of primary interest are the Hemoglobin (HGB), Hematocrit (HCT), red blood cells (RBC or Erythocytes), white blood cells (WBC or Leukocytes, and Platelets (PLT).

A urinalysis is used to determine the level of different proteins as well as the possibility of calcium being excreted in the urine. One protein known as M Protein helps to track status of MM and how the patient may be responding to treatment. A "spike" in this protein is a strong signal of presence of MM.

Because MM acts to break down bone structure, imaging is very important. The usual tests include a complete bone survey which is basically an x-ray approach, magnetic resonance imaging (MRI) and computerized axial tomography (CAT scan or CT scan). Each of these will show the bone structure somewhat differently and enable your doctors to get a better picture of what's happening to you.

Another type of image is the PET (positron emission tomography) scan. When this type of scan is done you first receive an injection of a small amount of radioactive substance which is administered with glucose. The cancerous cells suck up more of the glucose and show up as hot spots in the images, giving the doctors a better idea of just where the problems may be and the extent of them. Some providers may order up all these types of scans since each has its value.

A test called a bone marrow biopsy is used to measure the population of diseased cells in your bone marrow. There are usually two steps to this test. Aspiration takes out a bit of the liquid marrow, while the biopsy removes a small sample of the actual bone itself. The usual point of contact is the hip area, and the procedure is easily done right in the doctor's office with slight discomfort.

There are other tests that may include a "labeling" analysis which is done by the Mayo Clinic, determination of presence of Bence-Jones protein or studies to determine chromosome abnormalities such as a chromosome-13 deletion. New tests and markers are being developed in the race to find a way to quickly diagnose MM, determine the status or progression of the disease and suggest the best possible intervention from the many which are currently available.

MM does remain a disease which is enigmatic. Enigmatic in that there is no such thing as each patient at a similar point reacting in the same way to identical interventions. Enigmatic in that the same treatment which proved invaluable to Patient A, may be of little or no benefit to Patient B.

The fact that you are reading this book strongly suggests that you or a loved on is now diagnosed as having MM. We're past the early warning signs which can easily be misread, and now the urgent fight is to figure out what this MM thing is all about, and what to expect as the weeks melt off the calendar.

WHAT'S IT ALL ABOUT?

MM is not an easy disease to understand. The most basic definition is that it is a process in which deformed blood cells start to multiply without any controls on their production. These cells generally inhabit the bones of the patient where their presence causes damage. As they grow they play vampire and need to suck your blood to stay alive. To do so they start to create new blood supply lines, which you don't need.

The effect of this overgrowth plus the creation of new small blood vessels in the bones starts to break down the bones themselves. As the bones break down calcium is released into the blood stream and your kidneys attempt to get rid of as much of it as they can, along with excess protein. This is analogous to the termites destroying the dwelling, which they have invaded.

This over-simplification of the process of MM is not the complete story by any means. There are various types of myeloma and they range from a myeloma which requires no treatment other than careful monitoring, to the most severe which requires dramatic and immediate intervention.

You will hear the doctors refer often to a MM Stage. There is a classification table developed by Doctors Durie and Salmon that is commonly used to classify patients. Stage-1 refers to patients with a low cell mass of myeloma cells and who have a hemoglobin value greater than 10, with calcium values equal to or less than 12 milligrams per deciliter, with fewer than two or no malignant bone tumors, and a low production rate of M protein.

Jumping ahead to Stage-3, that is defined as patients who have a much higher myeloma cell mass and in addition to all of the conditions defining Stage-1 also have ONE or more of these symptoms; hemoglobin value less than 8.5, calcium value more than 12, advanced lytic bone lesions (tumors), or a high M protein production rate.

And Stage-2 is basically defined as patients who exhibit some symptoms but who don't fall specifically into Stages 1 or 3, but whose myeloma cell mass is in the mid-range. Each stage can then be sub-divided into Class A or B with Class A being those who have fairly normal kidney functions as shown by a serum creatinine value of less than 2 milligrams per deciliter or Class B being those whose levels are greater.

A newer classification system is now being used by many centers and it is the ISS (International Staging System) which is simplified so that Stage I = B2M (beta-2 microglobulin) <3.5 and albumin 3.5; Stage II = B2M <3.5 and albumin <3.5, OR B2M 3.5 to <5.5; and Stage III = B2M 5.5 or more and regardless of albumin.

There is also an International Prognostic Index (IPI) which is often referred to as CRAB because the index looks for problems with (C) calcium elevation, (R) renal problems, (A) anemia and/or (B) bone lesions.   When found along with monoclonal protein in blood or urine and monoclonal cells in the bone marrow this roughly approximates the Durie-Salmon Stages 2 and 3.

You will find simple definitions of medical terms and how to decipher the blood and urine analyses reports in the glossary.

You will hear of MM referred to by Classification as well as Staging. The least destructive situation is one in which you have been diagnosed with monoclonal gammopathy of undetermined significance (MGUS) and this is a situation where some monoclonal cells are determined to be present but there are no other symptoms and no treatment is indicated at the time.

That's the good news.   However, 10% to 15% of patients may develop MM over the course of time and treatment will be needed.

Smoldering multiple myeloma (SMM) patients generally do not show renal failure, nor do they have anemia, hypercalcemia or lytic bone lesions.   But, they do show some M protein production and/or have bone marrow plasma cells equal to or more than 10%.   SMM is also referred to at asymptomatic myeloma.   These patients are watched carefully and treatment is usually not commenced until the disease progresses.

Indolent multiple myeloma (IMM) refers to patients who do have a few small bone lesions but whose M protein production is stable and who have, perhaps, only a mild anemia.   These patients must be reviewed every 3 months with treatments started when the disease starts to progress.

And the big gorilla of the Classifications is symptomatic multiple myeloma (MM) where a patient shows M protein in blood and/or urine, malignant bone marrow cells greater than 30% of the sample and may also have anemia, renal failure, hypercalcemia, or lytic bone lesions. This is classic MM and demands immediate treatment.

MM affects the body in several ways. Perhaps the most obvious is the attack on the bones. As the diseased cells increase in population they show up as soft spots or holes in the bones. These are called osteolytic lesions or more commonly bone tumors. These damaged areas make your bones much more susceptible to breakage from falls, over-exertion, or may even produce bone fractures just by breaking down the bones. It is very common for a MM patient to quickly lose several inches of height. This may occur over a period of a few weeks, not years.

A couple of other critters come into play. Osteoclasts are cells that act to break down old and worn out bones so that osteoblasts can build new bone. This is the mechanism by which bones regenerate. However, in MM the production of osteoclasts is increased, the osteoblasts get outnumbered, the bones do not regenerate and bone destruction is accomplished. As the bones break down calcium is released into the blood and the dangerous condition known as hypercalcemia can occur.

Your blood cells are formed in your bone marrow. As myeloma cells take over, they inhibit the production of other cells. Lower production of white blood cells raises risk of infections.

Concurrently, lower red blood cell counts result in anemia commonly associated with MM. Fewer platelets interferes with proper blood clotting in the event of an injury; while the higher M protein and light-chain proteins associated with the MM may cause the blood to thicken.

If the blood gets too thick it can impair circulation in the kidneys. Also, the hypercalcemia overtaxes the kidneys which can't excrete it all and often causes the patient to go into dehydration. Care givers need to be alert to the signs of dehydration and make certain the patient gets plenty of fluids; unless some kidney problem prompts your physician to advise otherwise. Few of us are equipped to handle giving our patients an intravenous infusion at home. So if dehydration is present let your doctor know and if you can't get relief for your patient right away get him/her to the hospital.

The objective of this book is not to turn you into a doctor. Most doctors don't know much about this disease unless they specialize in blood disorders or cancers. What you need to understand is that this is a VERY serious and VERY confusing disease. Rounding up these blood bandits is like trying to eliminate all the terrorists in the world. Every patient is different. The disease will progress differently in different patients and respond differently to standards of care.   If there is one thing that is true when discussing MM, it is that all generalizations are wrong.

TREAT ME, PLEASE

Most of us would probably agree that as we wade through the description of this disease when advised of status by the doctor, what we really want to know is What Are we Going to Do About It. How do we treat this invader from inner space.

There are three basic approaches which are radiation therapy, chemotherapy and stem cell transplant. In addition to the Big Three there are alternative therapies, salvage therapies and supportive therapies. A most important thing to know is that as this book is being written at the start of 2004, that there are new advances being made on a very fast-track basis and that no book could possibly be fully up to date. Discuss possibilities with your doctor which may include recently approved therapies and some that are in clinical trials that you may want to be a part of.

If the MM is advanced and bone damage exists your doctor may order radiation therapy to start at once. Low dose radiation can be used as a pain reliever or to ward off possible injury to the spinal cord. High dose radiation is finely targeted use of high-energy rays to kill off the diseased cells where they are doing serious damage. If we go back to the termites again, this is to eradicate some nests where they are known to exist. If chemotherapy is a shotgun approach which goes to the entire body, then radiation is a rifle approach aimed at specific targets. It is also sometimes used in association with stem cell transplants.

Radiation therapy is done on a large, flat, cold and uncomfortable table with a giant x-ray type of machine moving around your body. The locations for the radiation will probably have been mapped out on your body with a somewhat indelible marker by the radiologist. Using these targets a computer model is created which will control the delivery of the radiation in the sessions which follow. Radiation may take place as many times as the doctors feel is necessary to kill off the cells without doing too much damage to the patient. Once the computer driver model is finished it is used in each session. Patients may experience nausea and quite often will experience a burning sensation or rash around the points of radiation. These will go away in due course.

Chemotherapy is what most of us become familiar with and it refers generally to the use of drugs to systemically attack the myeloma cells. Chemo (as it is usually called) may be by infusion or taken orally. And, there is not ONE chemo.

There are quite a few accepted standard regimen for chemo and others which are now under study. The dosages are variable within each type of chemo depending on the extent of damage experienced by the patient, the patient's ability to withstand the side effects of the therapy, and whether or not a stem cell transplant may be planned for the patient. Most MM patients will undergo chemo, which may take a few months or may extend for many months.

Quite often your doctor will suggest that you have a port installed. The procedure is done in the outpatient or short-stay section of a hospital and involves the installation of a tube which runs from a place on the upper portion of your chest, into the superior vena cava or other large vein. The port is installed just under your skin and the suture line is no more than an inch and hardly visible. Women who are concerned should know it usually lies just about under the bra strap line so it will not show in most clothing.

The port is basically an on-ramp to the highway system called veins. It allows medication to be infused without turning your arms into pin cushions, and it can also be used to draw blood when required for some blood tests. To access the port your care provider will simply feel for the location of the port, insert a needle which is nothing more than getting a shot in your arm, and then get the port ready by purging it to clean it and prepare it for the medication. The needle has a connection device at the end of it which then permits your chemo solutions to be hooked up to it.

Once the port is opened you are usually made to be at ease in a comfy chair while a bag containing a saline solution is hung on a device next to you and hooked up to your port. The saline is just a cleansing and diffusing agent and also helps to keep you hydrated. The smaller bag will contain the specific medications to be infused. The infusion involves no discomfort and depending on what protocols are being followed may take from 15 minutes to more than two hours. Bring a book to read or crosswords or just lie back and watch the TV if they have one.

When the infusion is finished your provider will then purge the port once again to clean it and you are done until the next visit. The cleansing of the port is very important because just as an exit ramp from the highway is sometimes the scene of an accident when a driver tries to use it for an entrance ramp, the port is an expressway for infection if not kept clean. Not to worry, your providers know what to do and they will keep it healthy for you.

The port is often referred to as a Port-Cath because it attaches to a tube (catheter) into the vein. It will stay in until it is no longer needed and when that happy day arrives it is a quick visit back to the outpatient section to have the surgeon remove the port and catheter. After the first few days you won't even know it's there, nor feel anything.

Orally administered chemo is simply the process of ingesting the meds as fluids or pills. When you get chemo it is typically given in cycles with a rest and recovery period between them. It's the side effects of chemo that are the stuff of horror stories. We'll discuss them in the next section.

Doctors tend to stay with the therapies with which they are most familiar and which they have seen work the best for their patients. By nature, many are hesitant to embrace newly emerging techniques, although in the most severe cases they'll try anything on the basis that even if it doesn't help it probably won't hurt.

The objective of chemo is to kill off the myeloma cells throughout the body and therefore it is the blood which circulates through you that is used to carry the medications to the culprits. Here is where we bog down a bit. New combinations of chemo are being developed all the time. Take this overview as only a terminology primer and not a medical treatment treatise. Discuss with your doctor alternatives in chemo or other therapies and learn what is in store for you. Remember that doctors love to speak in code that we mere mortals have trouble understanding. But we'll give you some of them here. **Caution: this is NOT intended to be a complete list, nor to discuss fully every aspect of any medication, or to include all possible side effects.** As with almost any medication if you were to read all the possible side effects you would find that most of them could cause just about anything you don't want to have happen.

A common chemo approach is called **VAD** and that is an acronym for Vincristine, Adriamycin and Dexamethasone. Vincristine is a clear fluid which is infused. It interferes with the growth of the cancerous cells. It makes you urinate more so you will want to drink plenty of fluids. And this is one of those meds which can cause constipation as well as hair loss. The Adriamycin is also used to attack the cancerous cells but this one can produce nausea and vomiting. And Dexamethasone (Decadron or "Dex") is a cortisone like med which is used to relieve swelling, redness, itching and other problems and as a steroid they are used to build strength. Because the Dex can lower resistance to infection be alert for signs such as fever, sore throat, coughing or sneezing.

MP stands for melphalan and prednisone therapy. Melphalan interferes with the growth of the cancer cells which are then destroyed by other means. It can be infused or be given as pills. It lowers your resistance so stay away from people who are ill, don't get any immunizations without first discussing with your doctor, and avoid anybody who has recently taken oral polio vaccine. Since it can lower white blood counts and platelets you want to stay away from anybody who is sick. You should be very careful not to get any skin lacerations and do not touch your eyes or pick your nose unless you have just washed your hands. Men should consider using an electric razor. Some doctors will advise to refrain from using toothpicks or mechanical toothbrushes. Prednisone is another corticosteroid which acts a lot like Dex, described above.

TD stands for thalidomide and Dexamethasone therapy. Yes, this is the thalidomide which caused those outrageous birth defects so many years ago. In recent years doctors have learned that this drug acts to inhibit the growth of blood vessels. The same action that caused such fetal development problems in the late 1950's and early 1960's, also acts to give hope to those who battle MM. It is a VERY closely controlled drug which is taken in pill form. Be sure to follow your doctors dosing instructions to the letter. Inasmuch as it will really make you drowsy most doctors tell you to take this before retiring for the night. You can't drink alcohol and take this med. In fact, make sure you clear with your doctor ANY med you take. He should have a complete list of all medications you use, including daily maintenance drugs and vitamins, and whenever you make any changes in that list he needs to know. See the section on keeping medical records.

While we're discussing thalidomide and the effect it can have for pregnant women, keep in mind that any patient with special conditions such as being of child bearing age, pregnant, nursing, or any patient with any other pre-existing conditions needs to make certain that the doctor knows all about it. Some meds can also aggravate conditions such as allergies.

D is just for plain Dex therapy. Usually given as tablets, or sometimes as an infusion on day one, followed by taking as many as 10 of these pills on days 2, 3 and 4, then a rest interval and resume the routine again.

C weekly refers to cyclophosphamide. Cyclophosphamide is another drug which attacks the cancer cells. It can cause bladder problems so most patients are told to take it in the morning, to urinate frequently, to drink up to 3 quarts of fluid a day. It often causes nausea, vomiting and loss of appetite. But then, many of the chemo drugs are going to cause these problems. It's all a question of what will work better for your case. This one is not one of the more friendly medications so be certain to have your doctor go over all possible side effects and some which may not manifest themselves until some years later. Cyclophosphamide is generally administered along with prednisone.

Velcade (bortezomib) is a newly approved drug which acts to kill off cancer cells. It is given by injection and used usually with patients who have not responded well to prior therapies.

ABCM refers to using a combination of Adriamycin, cyclophosphamide, melphalan and adding BCNU. BCNU refers to a drug also known as Carmustine and this also is used to kill off cancer cells. This one is given by injection. And, like so many of these type of drugs may cause nausea, vomiting, coughing or other side effects.

VBMCP refers to using a combination of Vincristine, BCNU, melphalan, cyclophosphamide and prednisone, each of which is detailed above.

VMCP/VBAP refers to using Vincristine, melphalan, cyclophosphamide and prednisone or Vincristine, BCNU, Adriamycin and prednisone. Each is detailed above.

dVD is not a video disc. It refers to using a reduced dosage of Dex together with Vincristine and liposomal doxorubicin (Doxil). This is given by injection. Doxil is also a med designed to kill off cancer cells. Be aware that this med will cause urine to turn red and you need to know this is not a discharge of blood. This will dissipate in a few days. Like some of the others, expect hair loss with this one.

The chemo procedures noted above are some of the more common ones. Remember that new drugs are on the fast track for FDA approval as this is being written.

When a patient has relapsed after treatment or has failed to respond to initial treatments the doctors may resort to what is known as Salvage Therapies. These almost always involve high doses of Dex with other meds mentioned above. Here are a few of the combinations.

CVAD stands for VAD combined with cyclophosphamide. Hyper CVAD just stands for higher levels of these meds.

MTD is a combination of melphalan, thalidomide and dexamethasone

TD as referred to above is also used in salvage therapies.

EDAP refers to some you haven't seen before. This is a combination of etoposide, dexamethasone, ara-C and cisplatin. Etoposide acts to slow the creation of cancerous cells. It often brings on nausea, vomiting, thinning of hair, stomach pain, appetite/taste changes and bowel changes. Ara-C is a drug called Cytarabine and is used to confuse the cancer cells since they think it is a nutrient they need but it really deprives them of growth factors. To the list of side effects you can add numbness or tingling of the extremities.

DT-PACE consists of 6 chemotherapy drugs (Dexamethasone, Thalidomide, CisPlatin, Adriamycin, cyclophosphamide, and etoposide) and is usually given to those patients who have not previously responded well. It is an emerging alternative therapy.

Finally, some doctors may employ thalidomide or cyclophosphamide alone as salvage therapy.

There are some other therapies referred to as Supportive which are designed not to attack the cancer cells, *per se*, but to help overcome the various side effects and problems of the disease. Some of them are described below, but the list is really somewhat endless depending upon your specific needs and the doctors recommendations.

To strengthen your bones the doctor may prescribe bisphosphonates such as Aredia or Zometa. These drugs are usually given by infusion and act to interfere with the termites called osteoclasts and they help to kill off some cells and inhibit more growth. One principal difference between the two drugs is that Zometa is a much faster infusion. The main side effect concern with either drug is kidney damage, so your doctor will want to carefully monitor your creatinine levels.

To help you deal with feeling so tired all the time, your doctor may want you to have Procrit, Epogen or Aranesp. These help your bone marrow to make more red blood cells and hemoglobin. These will substantially help improve the quality of your life while undergoing treatment as you should feel stronger and more alert with these.

Those patients who have very low white cell counts may also be put on meds to stimulate the production of them, such as Neupogen, Neulasta or Leukine. The main reason for using these types of drugs is to build up your resistance to infection.

If your bone pain is substantial it must be dealt with promptly. The objective is not to have pain that you can tolerate, but to make you pain free if possible. To that end you may be referred for surgical repair of injured bones. It may sound like something from outer space but they can really go in and insert a balloon in the vertebra which is then filled with a cement and this helps to restore the intervertebral space. This procedure is called kyphoplasty. A similar procedure without the balloon uses cement to repair the fractured bone in place.

A specialist can also use epidurals to alleviate extreme pain. This procedure which is commonly used in childbirth, involves the injection of anesthetics deep into the affected area and may take 3 to 6 sessions to bring about substantial relief.

It can be performed in an outpatient clinic or even in the office of a specialist who has the appropriate equipment on site..

In addition to all the above you will hear much about clinical trials for which you may be eligible. After testing on lab animals a new drug or therapy has to be tested on humans before it can be certified for general use. You'll hear the trials referred to as protocols. A protocol is just a detailed plan of who is desired as a subject and exactly how the plan will be administered. They may be a double blind (in which case you doctor will not know if you are in the control group or not) or they may be open. Usually there are two groups. The test group receives the new treatment and the control group receives the accepted current treatment that is sought to be superceded by the newly developed one.

Clinical trials are very important because without them there is no assurance that the information provided by the pharmaceutical company will actually produce results in use. But they are not for everyone. Such a trial may be organized by a cooperative research group, or a specific hospital, or other entity working with the medication under investigation. You may hear of a clinical trial being referred to as in a specific Phase.

A Phase 1 trial is a small group of patients who take different doses or methods of delivery. It is used to test the safety and dosage of the drug. In Phase 2 trials they use a larger group and test drug safety and efficacy by having two or more groups where one group gets the drug and others get the standard therapy or a placebo. In Phase 3 trials you find large scale studies with patients randomly selected to be on or off the drug without control of selection by the physicians. Occasionally you will hear of a Phase 4 trial which is after the drug is approved for use and is designed to study long term effects, sometimes among specific age groups.

Before you consent to go into such a trial you need to know everything about it and it must be explained to you in detail. The pharmaceutical company and/or the organizers will usually require you to sign an agreement by which they will pay you a pittance, you will not have to pay for the therapy, and you and your spouse will be releasing them from any and all liability for any and all damage. If your condition is such that nothing is working for you then you may have nothing much to lose. Otherwise, proceed with caution so that any consent you may give is truly an **INFORMED** consent. If you don't fully understand anything ask them to explain it in plain English.

The ultimate therapy is often a stem cell transplant. This procedure is utilized for more than 4,000 patients each year with significant success. The purpose of a stem cell transplant is to regenerate healthy blood cells after high dose chemotherapy has been utilized. Inasmuch as chemotherapy is a shotgun approach it does kill off many healthy cells as well as the diseased cells. Therefore, the transplant is used to help correct this deficiency.

A stem cell is a base cell which develops into either a red blood cell, a white blood cell or a platelet. The red blood cells are the ones which carry oxygen throughout your body. The white cells are the ones which carry the immunizing protection for your body and the platelets are things which help your blood to clot when you are bleeding. The stem cells are a very small percentage of all cells in your bone marrow.

Ordinarily stem cell transplants (SCT) are more effective when done earlier rather than later in the treatment and with patients who are fairly strong and don't have significant damage to their liver, kidneys, lungs or heart. While stem cell transplants may come from donors they are most often done by autologous transplantation.

An autologous procedure is one in which the cells are harvested from the patient and stored for reintroduction at a later date. The harvesting procedure is usually done before any high dose chemo is utilized, and the cells are kept frozen for use at a later date. This procedure involves the least risk of infection and rejection.

An allogeneic transplant is one where a donor who is usually a close relative is used, and providing the donor's cells match up as the same tissue type as the patient, the procedure is otherwise the same as autologous. The synergenic transplants refer to donors who are identical twins of the patient.

Regardless of the type of transplant, there are two sources of the cells. Sometimes the cells are extracted from bone marrow but more frequently they are extracted from what is called peripheral blood. Peripheral blood is drawn from veins and this technique is much less painful for the donor and also yields a better supply of stem cells. PBSC refers to Peripheral Blood Supply Cells.

A stem cell transplant is not a cure for MM. It does provide a complete response for about a third of the patients, of whom about half of them will experience a relapse within five years.

Obviously the picture is not as good for those patients who do not experience the higher level of response from the treatment.

SIDE EFFECTS

If it is true that no two patients follow the same path through MM then it may also be true that your reactions and experiences during your treatment may also be somewhat unique. Most common complaints include fatigue and nausea. Yet, the very same procedure or drug which may produce extreme nausea for one patient will produce no such response in another. The objective is to minimize or eliminate annoying, or even life-threateneing, side effects so that the patient experiences as little discomfort as possible.

The nausea experienced while taking the meds is a very common experience and fortunately there is an extensive arsenal of drugs with which this problem may be attacked. Phyllis was plagued with nausea for more than a year and the doctors tried more than a dozen different remedies. One group of doctors wiped their hands of the matter and just said she needed to see a gastrointestinal (GI) specialist. Another group did actually go many steps further and ordered up injections and infusions which helped to lower the level of the nausea while in the throes of chemo. More than a year into the disease, she was still relying on Ativan, which is taken orally and Carafate which is used to coat the stomach and esophagus to reduce the feeling of acid reaction or GERD (Gastroesophageal reflux disease). In her case she took the Carafate before every meal and at bedtime, and used the Ativan during the day when the nausea reared its annoying head.

Nobody wants to go around with a pocket or purse full of pills, or be tied down to counting out pills into little daily dosage containers. But, if the pills are going to help you it's better to put up with the discomfort of dragging them around with you than the discomfort of the symptoms they may help to rid you of. The point is that what works for one patient may be entirely different than what works for you. If the first prescription isn't giving you relief then let your doctor know right away and move on to another, and another, and keep trying until you find what may be of help.

In Phyllis' case, she did actually get to a GI and had an endoscopy and the good news was that they found nothing wrong. The bad news was that they found nothing wrong which might have accounted for the persistent nausea. One curious problem that nobody seemed to have any answer for, is that she seemed to develop a lactose intolerance which had never been present before. If you find that you have an almost immediate reaction after eating cottage cheese, ice cream or other milk products, then just delete them from your diet for a while and see if the problem diminishes. You can find plenty of other treats that don't contain lactose.

Fatigue is another huge problem for MM patients. Some of it is a reaction to the pharmaceuticals with which you are being treated, or it may be a reflection of lower red blood counts. Some may be due to the amount of energy that you have to expend just to accomplish some daily chores which you never even thought about before the MM appeared, and some may be a psychological reaction to the terrors with which you are dealing on a daily basis.

If you're tired and really wiped out and your body tells you that it wants to rest, the best advice is probably to respond by resting. While you are at rest your body can spend its energy on trying to get better without worrying about spending it on doing things that your care givers can do for you. You may find that you spend days when you hardly get out of bed. As you lay there with the insipid TV yakking at you, just console yourself by thinking of the better days to come. By all means, make sure your doctor knows you are wiped out. They can't respond to problems they don't know about, and don't worry about annoying the doctor. You'll be speaking with his nurse in most cases.

When you are in the fatigued mode you need to be extra careful about such things as walking down stairs, picking things up from the floor, carrying liquids or trying to drive a car. Let somebody else do these for you. Unfortunately there are few pharmaceutical interventions to get rid of fatigue. You get rid of it by getting rid of the other stuff that is causing it, and rest is the first remedy.

If your MM has produced bone lesions you may experience pain, usually in the spine, hips or shoulders. Your doctor will have extensive images taken to ascertain the location and extent of any skeletal damage. But, the objective in pain management is pain eradication. It may not be possible to achieve total relief, but you have a right to try to be pain free and that in itself will also help deal with the fatigue. Depending on the nature and extent of the pain there are a wide array of palliative meds ranging from simple acetaminophen to fairly high dose narcotics, injections, infusions, and trans-dermal opiate patches which you change every few days. If one approach doesn't do it for you ask them to try another. And another.

Diet changes are commonplace. By way of illustration I will again refer to my beloved wife. She is a woman who loved a glass or two of wine. Since she has been treated for MM it tastes like gutter swill to her, even though I swear that I buy the best wine that you can get in a 5-liter box. We used to joke that she ate so much salad that every rabbit had moved out of our neighborhood. Since the MM set in she has eaten perhaps 3 salads in a year. She loved asparagus, fish and some other foods that just no longer ring her chimes. If it doesn't appeal to you or tastes weird, just give it a pass. There's a good chance the taste buds may come back at a later time. For the time being, if you have to live on instant cream of wheat and blue boxes of mac and cheese, then so be it. Better to get some food into you that you can stomach (no pun intended) than to add hunger to your list of problems.

On that subject you may find that your eating times may be quite different than before. You may go along in the day without feeling hungry and all of a sudden your stomach starts growling to send food down NOW. OK, just do it. Who cares if you are dining at 11 AM or 11 PM? Keep some instant snack foods around such as saltines, canned beverages, peanut butter, etc. If you're going out, make sure you have them in the car with you.   And when away from the car take them with you.

Many patients get the shakes.   Not from McDonalds, but from Dexamethasone.   You may see you handwriting become almost illegible, you may have trouble handling pills, turning small knobs, using tools. Women may find they can't get their bra hooks into place because of the shakes as well as discomfort of reaching behind them.   These will usually pass when the drug has been out of your system for a while.

The more serious problem is peripheral neuropathy (PN) which may be associated with one or more of the medications used in chemotherapy, or just attributable to the MM.   This is the tingling in the extremities, more commonly the toes but often the hands and legs. The tingling is like when you fall asleep with your hand in a strange position and you wake up with what is known as paresthesia. Don't just sit around quietly if this starts. Get on the phone to your doctor right away, because PN may or may not be temporary. In more extreme cases it produces a numbness so that a patient can't feel pressure nor temperature changes.   It puts you in a position where you can hurt yourself without even knowing that you've done so.   Your doctors may be able to adjust your meds to reduce and/or eliminate this PN.

If you are going through chemo you will almost certainly lose your hair. Think of it not as a curse but as a badge of courage that sets you apart from and above the rest of us. Lost hair will grow back. Lost lives will not. A friend of my wife's who is a hair stylist did her a huge favor. She trimmed Phyllis' head down at the very start of the chemo so that she'd not have to go through the agony of waking up and finding large clumps of her hair on the pillow and sheets. This therapeutic approach may not work for everyone, but if you can deal with it you may find that you feel a lot better by planning ahead, having control, and avoiding the inevitable. You'll also have more time to select a wig you like, get a few head scarves and get used to it while you're still feeling more like yourself. By the way; what works for the gals here may also be a big help for men who have MM. And if you are concerned about how your disease impacts on your care givers and family members this way of dealing with the inevitable hair loss may also be a lot easier for them to handle than seeing you go through the distress of the adjustment over many days.

Your doctors will watch your blood counts closely because you may develop anemia which is associated with low levels of red blood cells, or neutropenia which is a decrease in white blood cells which fight off infections.   If your platelet count is low you may find that you are more susceptible to getting black and blue marks as the platelets facilitate blood clotting.

Headaches are also often reported and at times they can be severe.   These are often considered just part of the course and are treated with the usual OTC remedies; except that aspirin and NSAIDs such as ibuprofin are generally not used because of potential for kidney damage.

Constipation and diarrhea can both bedevil a patient.   And either can be very debilitating.   If you are experiencing either of these it is most likely due to the medications and the interactions of several of them.   By trial and evaluation you and your doctors should be able to find a recipe that works for you to control either.

THE DRUG SCENE

In your travels through the Myeloma Maze you will encounter a host of drugs including Thalidomide, Dexamethasone and dozens of others. No list or overview of drugs could be fully inclusive nor accurate for all patients since there are new drugs coming on the market, newer drugs still in clinical trials and different combinations of drugs being prescribed for the unique needs of each patient. You can get up to date information as to usual side effects, applications, and dosage from the various manufacturer's websites, the National Cancer Institute, the International Myeloma Foundation, the Multiple Myeloma Research Foundation and other reliable sites. One especially good site is at www.cancer.org

But, here again, let's be sure we understand that neither you nor I are going to play doctor. Sometimes the dosages prescribed by a physician for a specific patient's needs may seem significantly less than, or more than, the usual dosages mentioned in the web sites or the pharmaceutical company's literature. You may wish to ask your doctor why he or she is recommending the specified dosage. You have a right to ask and a right to know and if you don't fully understand the reply just politely ask for a clearer statement.

Here's some brief info on some of the more commonly used drugs. The usual brand name is **first** followed in parentheses by the generic name.

Adriamycin (doxorubicin hydrochloride) is given as an injection to kill of cancer cells

Anzemet (dolasetron mesylate) an anti nausea med which blocks the brain center which controls vomiting.

Aranesp (darbapoetin alfa) is like a natural hormone which stimulates red blood cell growth

Aredia (pamidronate disodium) acts to prevent bones breaking down and releasing calcium into the bloodstream. Usually given by infusion over a couple of hours.

Ativan (lorazepam) an antianxiety drug often used to help control nausea

Bactrim (sulfamethoxazole or sometimes called cortimoxazole) an antibiotic given by injection or as pills, keeps bacteria from reproducing

Carafate (sucralfate) may be pills or liquid. Used for ulcer patients but also to help ease digestive irritation during chemo

Celexa (citalopram hydrobromide) is an antidepressant which helps sharpen up mental processes by blocking serotonin uptake

Coumadin (Warfarin) a blood thinner usually given in low doses if a patient has a port installed

Decadron (dexamethasone) a steroid of many uses and commonly part of a chemo regimen

Diflucan (fluconazole) an antifungal which interferes with cells getting nutrients to grow

Duragesic (fentanyl) is a transdermal narcotic patch used to help control chronic pain

Klonopin (clonazepam) is an antianxiety drug used to help control nausea

Magnesium Oxide may be ordered if your blood labs show you are low in magnesium. It is available without prescription OTC

Marinol (dronabinol) legal prescription form of marijuana to control nausea

Maxide (hydrochlorothiazide) a diuretic used to help reduce edema

Miralax (polyethylene glycol 3350) is used as a powdered laxative for some patients

MSIR (morphine sulfate instant release) tablets used to help with moderate to severe pain

Oncovin (vincrinsitine) given as injection to kill off cell growth

Prilosec (omeprazole) is used to treat acid-related stomach and esophagus problems by blocking the production of acid in the stomach.

Quadramet (samarium lexidronam) is a nuclear medicine which is used to relieve bone pain and and is taken up in the bone cancer area where it then gives off radiation to help kill off malignant cells

Revlimid is a more potent version of thalidomide which should be in wider use by 2006

Thalomid (thalidomide) interferes with growth of new blood supplies which the cancer cells need in order to continue to reproduce

Velcade (bortezomib) given by injection used mostly for patients who have not responded well to other therapies. It blocks release of growth factors

Vicodin or Lortab (hydrocodone/apap) is a pain reliever for moderate pain

Xanax (alprazolam) is an anti-anxiety drug which also serves as a muscle relaxant and may serve as a sleep aid

Zometa (zoledronate) inhibits cancer cells from growing in bones and dividing

Zovirax (acylovir) is an antiviral which interferes with the growth of viruses such as herpes and chicken pox

COMMON SYMPTOMS

The MM patient may experience an array of symptoms some of which may be of long standing and others may seem newly inflicted. Don't ignore symptoms. It may help to keep a diary, although you'll soon have many notebooks filled with paper that you'll find impossible to wade through. But, you must stay alert to changes within your body and you should not hesitate to inform your doctors and care givers of changes.

Pain is something that many MM patients have learned to live with. But, the objective in treatment is not to lessen pain but to eradicate it. If you have been diagnosed as having lytic lesions (bone tumors) and you start to have more skeletal pain in the same locations, or new pains in other bone locations then let your doctor know right away. If there is no external cause for the pain, such as an injury, he will want to get some images made to determine the cause.

Fatigue is common as a patient goes through treatment. And an occasional day when you just feel as if you wish you didn't even have to get out of bed, is not a big deal. For some of us it's hard to tell the difference among fatigue, depression and drowsiness.   Many of the drugs will cause drowsiness (somnolence) and you just feel like nodding off. Do it. It's your body's way of saying it wants more time to help rebuild.

Patients, just like their care givers, may experience depression or anxiety during the course of treatment. I'm not sure where depression ends and anxiety begins because the symptoms are often quite similar.   And there are some drugs which may be used to treat either of them.   Certainly being anxious over the disease and where it is taking you, can cause you to become depressed, especially if you've been in treatment for a considerable time and aren't seeing the positive progress you would like to see.   Discuss these problems with your doctor and if he is one of those who treat bodies but is less helpful in treating minds, don't hesitate to ask for a referral to a psychologist or psychiatrist.   MM is a tough trial, and you need to get the help you need wherever and whenever you need it.

On the subject of fatigue and depression, it's a puzzle since either may cause or feel like the other.   If you are fatigued for a long time you may find it depressing.   If you are depressed you may feel worn out and fatigued.   Blood work may show lower red cell and/or hemoglobulin counts and that may signal systemic fatigue. You can get a booster shot to help get you back up and running. But, that isn't going to do much for a psychological problem. On the other hand, there are drugs which are anti-depressants and anti-anxiety reliefs which may help you feel a lot better and give you the desire (if not the ability) to do more. My test is if you have the desire and mind-set to get up and get going and your body says "Forget it" then that's fatigue.

Nausea is a common problem for patients who have had chemo and may endure for a long time, even after heavy dose chemo has finished. It's annoying, depressing, enervating, and may indicate a problem which needs to be addressed by a gastro specialist. There are a host of products out there to help control nausea. Sometimes you can do it with over the counter products, but if that doesn't work there are medications you can take, and in severe cases an infusion may be ordered to get higher doses of the drugs into you in a controlled manner. Nausea may be related to the chemo, may be a symptom of GERD (gastro esophageal reflux diagnosis).

In addition to treatment with meds, mild nausea may be controlled by use of a Relief Band which is basically a small TENS (transdermal electro neural stimulator) machine worn like a wrist watch. It's most often used by pregnant women who are uncomfortable as they go about their daily chores, or by airline passengers who need help with in-flight nausea.

Acupressure may also help to relieve nausea. There's an area on the left leg about an inch below the kneecap and slightly to the distal (outer) side where gentle pressure applied by a care giver may help relieve nausea. If you visit an acupressure specialist have somebody closely observe the pressure points so that you can have them administer the relief at home. This point is described as 2 cun below the knee. A cun is a Chinese measure equal to the width of the middle joint of the patient's thumb. Another point is located 2 cun below the distal wrist crease on the patient's lower arm.

Loss of appetite is quite common, as is changes in taste. The appetite loss is probably related to how your body feels and your mental state, while the taste changes are certainly related to the medications. If all you feel like eating is plain spaghetti or macaroni and cheese, then you can get by on that for a while. You can also get cream of wheat in little instant packets which can satisfy the need to have some nutrition. As Phyllis went through MM she existed for months on mac and cheese and instant cream of wheat. The appetite will return, so don't worry about it as long as you get nutrition. Some patients who loved such things as salads or a glass of nice wine with a meal, may find that salad is a turn-off and the wine taste like poison. Don't worry about it. The taste buds may get back to normal later on, and when you start having the desire for your old favorites again you'll know you're on the mend.

Dizziness or loss of equilibrium is something you need to be wary of. In and of themselves they may not be that problematic, and they may certainly be directly related to some of the meds. But they can put the patient in danger of injury. You don't want to fall down, trip, or strike yourself against sharp edges. MM patients may have a very serious risk of skeletal fractures and damage and they certainly don't need extra surgery in addition to everything else they are dealing with. Also, there are many times when the immune system of an MM patient is compromised, so you don't want any injury which breaks the skin. Even if you just break the skin in a way that you normally would ignore or just cover with a bandage, stop what you are doing. Clean the wound, apply an antibiotic cream, then cover with bandage. If you bang your arms or legs against hard objects you may find that you produce a nice hematoma (black and blue area). This is because the blood thinners you may be taking make you so much more susceptible to this type of injury. Unless it is very large, increases in size or is otherwise painful, assume it will pass with time.

Reduced mental processing time may be the result of some meds and in extreme cases may be result of hypercalcification. Some of the medications interfere with the neural transmitters which send signals across the synapses of the brain. In plain language it just slows down one's mental processing. Somebody asks you a question such as "Do you want coffee or would you prefer tea?" Ordinarily you would respond instantly, but when your processing time is impaired they may stand there for a minute while you think about it and communicate. It's especially difficult for care givers who have to remind themselves to be patient. One other aspect of this phenomenon is that the patient probably ought not to drive since reaction times are impaired. This will pass. It does not mean that the patient is suffering from Alzheimers although that certainly can be a complication associated with the aging process for some patients.

Similarly many patients may find that they forget simple things such as where they last left their pills, or that their care giver explained something to them just the day before. Usually it is the short term memory that becomes temporarily impaired. They can still recall details of life experiences from years past. If you're the care giver and your patient loses himself in mid-sentence just bring him back to it when he is done with the discourse upon which he has embarked.

Shortness of breath and labored breathing may be symptoms of pneumonia or of other pulmonary problems. If the symptom is not relieved by just sitting quietly for a while, it needs to be reported to the physician. If this is commonplace on a daily basis when first arising for the day, just sit on the side of the bed for a minute or two before getting up to permit your body to adjust to the change. If still bothered, your doctor will want to get an image to rule out any infection, bleeding or other lung complications.

Care givers need to watch out for hypercalcification, which may be caused by the breakdown of bones done by the MM cells which then releases extra calcium into the blood stream and which overwhelms the kidney's ability to eliminate the calcium. Typically the patient will be dehydrated, be very somnolent, will move extremely slowly, if at all, and will be unable to verbally respond to simple questions or make a decision for himself. This is when the care giver has to make the decisions since the patient can not do so. If during office hours call the doctor immediately. If not, call 911 and get the patient to the hospital. Do not let dehydration persist, get fluids into your patient right away. The saline solution that they will hook up to him at the ER is just that; hydration.

PHYSICAL CHANGES

It is probably true for most of us that we go through several lives in our lifetime. With MM in the family that is very much the case. Life as it was before was a different life. The job at hand is now to deal with the life of treating the MM, and planning a life for the future with the MM.

The most obvious physical change for many patients is a loss of height caused by the breakdown of the vertebrae. This does not affect all MM patients, but when it does it can be difficult to deal with. Phyllis lost almost 4 inches of height in less than 3 months and it was a tough experience for her. But, as I got involved with the local support group I met others who had the same traumatic experience, including a man who had lost more than 12 inches of height in one year. While your own experience may seem a disaster, there are always others who have had it much worse. Keep your eye on the goal which is to improve, survive, and get on with living.

Those who go through chemo will usually suffer a loss of hair. For some older guys this is no big deal as all they had left was that fringe stuff. For women the case is not the same. The experience of waking up and finding big clumps of hair on your pillow and bedding can be terrible. We have a dear friend who is a hair stylist and she suggested that Phyllis allow her to closely trim her hair so that she would not have to go through the trauma of the hair loss. As a result, Phyllis picked the day it would be done, knew what to expect, had been fitted with a wig and never regretted having opted to take this step. It's one option and it's up to you.

MM is a very emotionally charged experience. When you start to read about it and talk to the doctors you learn that as of the date that this is written the disease is incurable and that the long term survival rates are pretty depressing. That happens to be true, but more progress has been made in the past few years than was made in the several decades preceding them. If you have to have MM, there was never a time which held out greater promise of long term survival with decent quality of life than exists today.

Notwithstanding that, it is very understandable that we start to feel anxious or depressed. Why did this happen to me? What did I do? How might I have prevented this? Who is going to care for those I love? How will I complete the things I wanted to do in my life? You are not alone. The answers are that nobody knows why MM strikes where it does. The disease is an equal opportunity attacker, although statistics suggest it is more prevalent among blacks, men and those over 65. Having said that, I've seen more women than men, more Caucasians, and plenty of patients under the age of 40. So much for statistics.

You did nothing that caused MM. It wasn't diet, smoking, use of drugs, or lifestyle. You could neither have foreseen the problem nor prevented it. All you can do is deal with it. Those you love who you are worried about caring for will repay that love with care for you as you fight the MM. It's almost incomprehensible to think that there are some people who can effectively fight MM on their own. Discuss your concerns with your doctors. Don't eschew the medications for relief of depression and anxiety. Take each day as it comes and make the most of every day. You'll get there, perhaps more slowly and with more effort than before, but you can still accomplish much.

You will probably experience anemia when your red blood cell counts are low. The red cells carry oxygen to all the rest of your body. You'll be sluggish, and have breathing difficulty. The doctors can give you a shot to boost your red blood cell count (RBC).   Your doctor may order a transfusion, or may give you an injection of Aranesp or similar drug. The anemia, itself, won't be a big problem.

You will want to stay away from activities which can put you at risk. MM patients aren't going to be found doing much skiing or playing tennis. If you've been a globe trotter you will find yourself staying closer to home and to medical care you can rely upon. Think of your energy supply like a debit card. Conserve it and spend it wisely because when you use it up there isn't any more until you recharge it. Many patients want to push themselves in activities because they are bored, or feel that they don't want their care giver to have to do everything for them, or perhaps that by doing some activity they are validating the concept that they are getting better.

Rubbish. If you are the patient and you overextend yourself you are just going to prolong your own recovery and put more work on your care giver's plate. Exercise and activity are good and you don't want to just sit in a chair all day and do nothing. Moderation is the key. When your body tells you it wants to stop, STOP! Better to rest now and go back to whatever it may be at a later time.

Sleep habits may change dramatically. Patients may find they want and need a nap in the morning and/or the afternoon. Some patients are zonked out during the day and just start to come around later in the evening when their care giver is about ready to drop from exhaustion. The story is just that when you are tired you need to sleep. When you aren't, you won't easily fall asleep without some more sleep inducing meds.

The same sort of situation occurs with eating times. You may be hungry an hour after you last ate. So have something to eat. You may want your supper at 4:30. So do it. You won't want to eat when you are not hungry but you need the nutrition; so when you are hungry go ahead and chow down. MM patients find their appetite may diminish so that those who would ordinarily destroy a 12 ounce steak, have trouble getting through a 4 ounce hamburger. The size of the meal is not important. What is important is that you get nutrition.

Your weight may fluctuate as much as 10 pounds in a week. Don't get crazy over it. You don't need to be on a diet at a time when you need to be building up your body. We've used a drink made from a protein whey powder which helps a lot on days when regular diet seems out of the question. You can buy a big jug of whey in the vitamin stores or even at Wal-Mart, and here's one recipe, although there are certainly many others or you can make up your own.

Use a blender and put in one cup of cranberry juice, one cup of high pulp orange juice, 2 or 3 scoops of the powdered whey and either a teaspoon of sugar or a packet of sugar substitute. Now blend the drink. To make it much thicker and greatly enhance the food value of the drink get some frozen strawberries and frozen peaches as well as some bananas. Add a cup of defrosted berries, a cup of defrosted peaches and break up one banana and place it in the blender with the other items, and grind it all up. It actually is good smelling, tasting, easy to get down, and very nutritious. We saved one of the 64 oz. cranberry juice jars and when we make the drinks we store them in one of those jars.

TELL ME MORE

So MM has entered your life.   You want information.   There's plenty of it out there.   You can start reading everything you can get your hands on and in the process it may seem like trying to shovel your way out of a quagmire.   I have said to many doctors that as far as MM is concerned I often feel as if the more I learn the less I know, and they understand completely where I'm coming from.

I told one friend who wanted to know what to do when he first heard about MM and my advice was to stay away from the internet for a while, and then to proceed with caution.   There are some great sites out there but there are also some that have been put up by people who just have something they want to peddle to you.   You don't need W. C. Fields pulling into town with a medicine man show. Just keep in mind that the internet is a gold mine, but it is also a gold mine surrounded by a mine field and you need to have a good idea where you're going to avoid problems.

There are quite a few really authoritative sites out there many of which are which I have listed in this section I would recommend starting out at International Myeloma Foundation, Multiple

74

Myeloma Research Foundation and National Cancer Institute and then branch out from these acclaimed and authoritative sites. The sites which are written primarily for physicians may well be unintelligible to you unless you happen to be one.

If you have a MM support group in your area you may find it a source of information, comfort and comaraderie. There are some very dedicated people involved in these groups, and it's always good to know that you are not alone on this journey.

If you live in a city where there is a MM symposium being held, I highly recommend that you try to attend. Both of the major research foundations hold these events in various cities and they bring in the top authorities to speak. Most of these physicians are very approachable and it's a lot easier to ask questions there than to get office time with them back at their hospitals.

Here are some of the top resources you may wish to contact. I have included both a web address and a phone number. Please note that if calling from outside North America, the 800 series area codes may not work but you can get a direct dial number at their website.

American Association for Cancer Research
www.aacr.org
215-440-9300

American Cancer Society
www.cancer.org
800-227-2345

American Instituite for Cancer Research
www.aicr.org
800-843-8114

M. D. Anderson Cancer Center
at University of Texas
www.mdanderson.org/care_centers/lymphoma/
800-392-1611

Association of Online Cancer Resources
www.acor.org
212-226-5525

Blood & Bone Marrow Transplant Info Net
www.bmtnews.org
888-597-7674

Cancer Care
www.cancercare.org
800-813-4673

Cedars-Sinai Medical Center
www.csmc.edu/5.html
310-423-4444

The Cleveland Clinic
www.clevelandclinic.org/myeloma/
216-445-6830

Dana-Farber Cancer Institute
www.dana-farber.org
866-408-3324

Gilda's Club Worldwide
www.gildasclub.org
917-305-1200

Hospicelink
www.hospiceworld.org
800-331-1620

International Myeloma Foundation
www.myeloma.org
800-452-2873

Leukemia & Lymphoma Society
www.leukemia.org
800-955-4572

Mayo Clinic
www.mayoclinic.com

MedlinePlus Dictionary of Medical Terms
from National Institutes of Health
http://medlineplus.gov/

Multiple Myeloma Association
www.webspawner.com/users/myelomaexchange/

Multiple Myeloma Research Foundation
www.multiplemyeloma.org
203-972-1250

Myeloma Institute for Research and Therapy
www.myeloma.uams.edu
888-693-5662

National Cancer Institute
www.nci.nih.gov
800-422-6237

National Marrow Donor Program
www.marrow.org
800-627-7692

Patient Advocate Foundation
www.patientadvocate.org
800-532-5274

THE BEST ROUTE TO TAKE

There is no single regimen which can be applied to all patients with MM. Often times the choice of alternative therapies is one of trial and error. Or perhaps it would be better stated as trial and evaluation.

We have all heard of the possibilities of bone marrow transplants. Actually there are very few bone marrow transplants being done today and they have been pretty much replaced by stem cell transplants, most of which are denominated as peripheral blood stem cell transplants, meaning the source is the least invasive possible.

Not all doctors will want to order a SCT and not all patients are good candidates for the procedure. It was thought that older patients would not benefit from the transplant. Up until 2000, Medicare would not pay for even one transplant, let alone a tandem (double) transplant. Today they will pay provided the patient has no serious impairment of heart, liver, kidneys or lungs and is in good enough general physical condition to withstand the procedure.

Patients who have smoldering myeloma or MGUS will not be receiving SCTs, and may not even be on low dose chemo. They may just be on "watch and see" regimen. As of 2004 the standard therapies remain chemotherapy, high-dose chemo, stem cell transplants, radiation and palliative care.

You may recall that in years past cancer patients flocked to Mexico to receive a treatment derived from apricot kernels. As of 2003 the news reported that people in Cuba were being cured of cancer by taking Escozul derived from the venom of the blue scorpion. Those avenues are still open although they have come under attack from the FDA as well as private foundations. Similarly you may find promoters of other novel "cures" outside the USA and the EU. Before you book your trip to the Caribbean or some other less controlled venue give some thought to this one question. If the people in the remote location have been obtaining credible results for many years as they claim, does it make sense that the dedicated investigators at home would not have taken up the challenge and moved to adopt a proven treatment, provided it could be proven. Proven is the controlling word.

Most of the MM specialists I know would give their right arm if they could find a cure for this disease. They are among the most dedicated physicians and researchers in the world. Don't make a decision in the closet. Talk to your MM doctors. If they are just dismissive of the novel approach, or say they know nothing about it, you can talk to another specialist. But, when all the talking and investigation is over, it's your life and you make the call as to whether or not you want to gamble. Obviously that decision may also reflect where you are in the progression of the disease, and what you may have to lose.

CARE GIVING

One of the most helpful things that a patient and care giver can do is to try to maintain a positive mental attitude. It isn't easy to do, and many days it's so hard to even care what's happening as you try to mentally dissociate from the problem.

MM is when you are going to truly appreciate the goodness of family and friends. Even though you may not want to call upon them for help, you will find that when they offer to do something for you the best thing to do is gratefully accept their offer. MM is not a short trip; rather it's a long and arduous journey through uncharted waters and you need all the help you can find.

Keep in touch with family and friends. Even on days when a patient may not feel that much like being on the phone, he or she will appreciate a note that may have arrived, the loan of a video tape, some photos that are sent, the loan of a book or maybe a some home-made soup or dinner entree.

If you are the care giver you will find that this is a full time job. If your neighbor wants to cut your grass for you, or shovel a walk through the snow, that's great. If friends want to come for dinner and want to bring the dinner, that's even better. Know that this is a balancing act. While the MM is always there, you will also have to find ways to put it into the back of your thoughts and get on with life to the extent that it is possible to do so.

And with this we come to the term, *Carpe Diem* which means simply, "Seize the Day." There are going to be lousy days, but deal with them secure in the knowledge that there are also going to be better days. And when you have those better days, get out and get going and do something enjoyable. A change of scenery, a change of activity, a change of diet are all good changes and for the patient and care giver, these little things can mean a lot.

If you're the patient and you're suffering and feeling terrible, know that there's nothing wrong with communicating that. Your tears are fully understandable and nobody will think the less of you for shedding them. On the other hand, if you're the care giver, try to shed those tears in the middle of the night when your beloved patient can't see or hear you. For you have to be both the tower of strength and the disciple of hope. Encourage your patient to move around, to walk, to exercise when he/she is able to do so. Keep pushing nutrition, and help organize the masses of medications and the diaries that will inevitably become the history of the journey.

Above all, if you are the care giver, do not let your patient retreat into a mental cave and hide from those who are concerned and who want to know and want to help. Try to make your own schedule flexible to accommodate your patient's needs and sometimes strange hours of wakefulness.

HOUSEKEEPING

You may find that many housekeeping changes will have to be made to accommodate your patient's needs. Most of them can easily be done.

Many patients may find that they need help walking. If the situation is severe a wheelchair may be required. In less severe circumstances a walker or a cane may suffice. Know that just because a MM patient may need a wheelchair at one time, does not mean that this is what life will necessarily be for all time. I can relate from our personal experiences that Phyllis went from being almost unable to walk, to a wheelchair, to a walker, to a cane, to being able to walk unaided in less than 5 months as her treatments progressed. The wheelchair lives downstairs in our home against the possibility it could be needed at a later date.

Most insurance plans will cover some durable medical goods such as wheelchairs, walker and lift chairs. If there's the slightest suggestion that some one of these would be of help for your patient, get them ordered and do not delay. Many insurors may try to deny coverage for durable medical goods, but get a letter of medical necessity from your doctor and start beating up on your insurance company. Most will accede to your needs when they know you are serious

One problem with walkers is that if you have both hands on the walker, how do you carry something else such as a cold drink or some snacks? You can easily attach a plastic shoe box to the front rail with wire or those plastic cable ties they use for computers. Then you can use the walker, carry what is needed and still fold it up easily..

One item you may need is a raised toilet seat for your patient. These are just white plastic appliances which can either be affixed semi-permanently to the existing toilet or simply set onto the bowl when required. If you have more than one toilet in your home, then get the type that is attachable since you can then designate that bathroom for your patient and others in the home may use the other toilets. This way your patient doesn't have to find the seat, put it in place and then use it. When you're hurting, the less bending and lifting you do, the better you may feel.

If the patient has suffered bone damage, especially vertebral, just taking a bath or shower can become a very arduous job. Start off by realizing that even though you may have bathed every day for the past 20 years, that if you don't do anything during the day other than sit in a chair trying to feel better, that you probably don't need to bathe as frequently.   If you have a walk-in shower stall you may want to make certain that you have a handrail installed if needed, and may need some kind of seating as many MM patients just don't have much energy for standing.   You can get a bench seat from a medical device company for $150 or you can get a plastic patio chair at Wal-Mart for $8, and either will work quite well.   If the $8 chair has no drain holes in the seat, just drill a few in the lowest part of the seat and it will work just fine.

Tripping and falling are constant threats.   In our home we had a good sized mat on the kitchen floor in front of the sink and counter.   We removed it.   In the bedroom we had a small Persian rug which we liked and it sat atop some other carpeting. We removed it for several months to get rid of any possible surfaces that could catch her foot.   If there are kids around, make sure the toys aren't left where the patient may have to walk.

We may aspire to reach for the stars, but if your back is hurting and if you have lost inches in height, you may find that those things on the top shelves are more difficult to get to.   You can easily reorganize your kitchen storage so that things the patient may want to get at are neither down at floor level nor stored over head.   Then stock up on the food items the patient is likely to want to eat on a moment's notice. If the patient may want to cook something simple for a snack there's nothing wrong with leaving a frying pan or saucepan out on the stove for him/her.   It's not likely that Martha Stewart will be dropping in to take pictures, is it? Just try to make things easy.

If you live in a two story home, you will want to make certain there is a hand rail on the stairs.   And if you are one of the last families without a cordless telephone you will want to buy one so that you can have it at hand wherever you may be.   When you do buy a phone if you can find the type on which you can turn off the ringer, that helps when the patient needs to nap and doesn't need to be awakened by a telemarketer.   If the care giver is busy working in another part of the house and the patient is in tough shape it helps to have an intercom system and/or some walkie-talkies.   The intercom stations are better since they can be set to monitor and won't require the patient to do anything to be heard.   You can find these kinds of intercoms at eBay, or even in stores selling baby supplies.   The walkies are available at any office supply store. Buy the cheapies as they aren't going to need to transmit very far.

Being a care giver is a matter of being there and caring. While nurturing may come more easily to women, it does require a little more thought for some men. Most of us haven't been conditioned to think in terms of what to make for dinner, especially when we just had lunch. We may be the masters of the VCR remote control, but we seem to have problems understanding the complexities of washing machines and vacuum cleaners. Rise to the occasion, guys. If she can learn how to handle that stuff, we're all Einsteins and we should be able to do so.

And that's why stocking up is so important. If you're using bottled water or ginger ale (for nausea) always buy what you need now; and then buy an extra case for later. You can store it in the garage or some corner of the house. Make sure you get an extra jug of laundry detergent, replacement collection bags for the vacuum cleaner, and keep extra soup, bread, butter, tea, and other edibles on hand. Some advance planning will save you so many extra trips to the grocery store and Home Depot.

Believe it or not there are some frozen entrees which are actually edible, although so many of them are not. Try one in the microwave. When you find one that the patient can stomach just get another one and toss it in the freezer. Otherwise toss it elsewhere.

Some of the supplies which may be required at some time by your patient may include flexible drinking straws, stack tables, extra pillows, a light weight blanket, extra cushion for the car, some of those seven-compartment pill organizers, a diary, an organizer or notebook. And, if the patient has experienced some bowel incontinence you will also want to have bed liners, panty liners, clean wipes and disinfectants at hand. They're all available at the drug store and if you need them you'll be glad if they're on hand. Constipation is a big problem for many patients. If you have never experienced the pain of not being able to evacuate your bowels then you really can't understand just how miserable it can be. If you've discussed it with your doctor he may have prescribed some laxatives. Most will work when they feel like it and stop working when they feel like it. Sort of like cell phones. Get a box of suppositories and just keep them on hand against possible need. You should also get a box of disposable surgical gloves, as you may occasionally need them.

Please buy some of those night lights that turn on when it is dark. You don't want a patient to get up in the middle of the night and trip on the way to the bathroom. Put one in the bathroom, one in the bedroom and another in the hall going towards the kitchen. Get a decent flashlight and some extra batteries. If you live in an area which is prone to power outages, make sure there's a flashlight in the patient's night stand, and another in a set place in the kitchen. You may need several of those seven-compartment weekly pill holders, and a small pill container that will fit easily into purse or pocket.

A lap table will come in very handy. These are the things the kids use in lower grades in some schools and are about 12 x 24 inches and usually have a bean bag attached to the underside. They'll provide a steady surface for a patient to eat from when he/she is more comfortable in a lift chair or a bed as opposed to sitting at the table.

WE NEED HELP NOW!

"I'm sorry, but you have called when we just don't bother to answer the phone. If this is an emergency, please hang up and call 911 . . . ." Don't you just hate those messages? Especially when they are preceded by an announcement which says "Our office hours are 8:30 AM to 5:00 PM. . ." and you're looking at your watch which says 9:15.

Especially in the big practices with quite a few physicians, the ladies at the front desk always seem to be engaged in everything other than responding to patients. Life is a series of trade-offs. You need them more than they need you. There are always plenty of patients. Look around the waiting room. In some practices the wait is so long that a few of them in the back rows have actually grown moss as they wile away the day reading old copies of National Geographic.

But, thanks to the insurance companies and the legal profession the practice of medicine today has become the practice of paper-shuffling and documentation and that's why it takes several non-medical personnel to support each physician. So they're a little late taking their phones off service. "Service" is the answer center that screens calls for them. So maybe they go on service a little early before lunch and come off service a little late, and then go on service at 4:30 when you know darn well they're all there until well after 5 PM. It's just part of the practice of medicine in contemporary America. Deal with it. Don't let the steam come out of your ears.

If you have a doctor who actually uses email and actually responds to it in person or through his aide, then use it. But, when you don't get a reply in a reasonable time, resort to the phone. It's not uncommon that his nurse or some administrator will have sick days or go on vacation and not bother to program an auto-reply email to advise you that they aren't really there. Naturally, nobody else will bother to read the email so you can sit in the dark. The same is true of voice mail. In many cases the person who answers the phone at the office hasn't a clue as to whether or not the person you are calling is actually there, alive and in person. So you get the ubiquitous voice mail. If no reply in a reasonable time, call again. Then call and ask if anybody has seen the person actually breathing and walking around. It helps to know if there's some chance the message actually got to somebody.

If you think that some medical practices can be frustrating to deal with, just try dealing with insurors, Medicare or Medicaid.   That's when you will start considering becoming an alcoholic, and you will be convinced that nobody ever answers a phone themselves, nor replies to anything. Keep at them. The wheel which squeaks gets the grease.

But, to be serious, ... if the patient has a problem that is different, that you are not certain how to deal with, or that you are seriously concerned about, then your patient needs attention and needs it NOW.   When a doctor's office is on service during the day there isn't much that will get done with your call until they come back on line. But, at night and on weekends there should be one of the doctors who is on call.

The fastest way to get through to the call center to get them to take a message is to press the button saying you are a doctor or hospital calling. This also happens to work pretty well with pharmacies, too.   You will listen to a seemingly endless message about how they will not refill narcotic prescriptions outside of office hours, and that you need to disconnect your caller ID, etc. When the human answers she will need the patient name, the doctor's name, the call back number and some indication of the problem.   This person you are speaking with is a telephone clerk and not a medical person so she isn't going to do anything other than forward your call to the doctor on call, or to his nurse or other assistant.

Most good services will tell you that if the doctor hasn't called within 20 minutes that you should call them back. That's because they may be using a pager or leaving a voice message on his cell phone. The really good services will also call you back in about a half-hour to ascertain that the doctor has called you. Keep your phone clear. If Aunt Sally calls, just tell her, "Later" and terminate the call.

But, when the condition is really serious such as a fall, inability to move, really hard time breathing, bleeding, or serious dehydration then that's when you need to just push 9-1-1 and get on with it. Depending on your home town's practices, the 911 operator will already know your address when she answers the call. She'll ask the problem, and then dispatch help.

We've had a few trips to the hospital with the 911 routine. In our community the standard practice is to dispatch both an ambulance and the fire department rescue squad. Twice I told the operator that they didn't need the whole fire department deal, but guess what. They showed up with sirens blaring. Neighbors loved it at 6 in the morning! This is a normal procedure and in the event a patient needed CPR or oxygen these are the folks who could respond fastest. In fact, if you are in a two story home, you'll be glad they are there to help get the chair or gurney down to the ambulance.

Don't assume the ambulance driver knows where you want the patient taken or even that they necessarily know how to get there. If your doctor practices at Hospital A, then barring some truly life-threatening situation in which every minute counts, you want to go to Hospital A, and not Hospital B which may be 2 miles closer to home. You need to tell the ambulance driver where you want them to go, and you may even want to ask if they know how to get there from where you are. Unless you have a friend or family member who is going to meet you at the hospital and bring you home later, you don't want to ride in the ambulance. Take you own wheels and follow the siren and red lights. It's a great way to get through the morning rush hour.

RECORD KEEPING

If MM is a journey through uncharted waters then the keeping of charts and records becomes of even greater importance. And, the care giver is the one who is going to have to organize and maintain those records. So the earlier you get organized the easier it will be when the days become more confusing.

Recommended supplies would be to get a 3-hole punch and a couple of ring binders at least 2 inch size. Don't bother with normal 1 inch size binders as you'll outgrow them in a month. At the back of this book you'll find some record keeping charts and forms which you can easily copy. Enlarge them to about 150% and they'll do just fine on standard 8.5 x 11 inch paper. Or use your computer to download from our storage at www.mydocsonline.com/pub/mmforms/dwnld.pdf where you can go directly to your computer and printer.

MEDICATION PRICE LOG - If you have insurance you probably have a maximum cap on the amount they will pay for prescriptions. You will blow through that in a flash. You will want to keep a log of what you pay for each prescription and where. Because, unlike some other countries with drug price controls, the retail drug business in America is a Wild West Show. You may find as much as a 50% price differential among major chain retailers. So you will have to play the game of always calling 3 stores to get prices and then deciding where to buy. Many chains will match prices, so just ask them. CVS and Walgreens will not, so they go to the "B" list. If you keep this log then you will know what you will expect to pay and can be watchful.

Keep in mind that most drugs have generic equivalents. Unless there's a good reason to require the branded drug, insist the druggist dispense the generic. Many of them fail to put on the label what the generic is substituted for, so tell them to be sure to do so. You may forget that alprazolam is really Xanax, lorazepam is Ativan, etc.

Play the generics game even with OTC (over the counter) items you may need. Dulcolax is bisacodyl. Look at the active ingredients info on the back of the box. Then pick up the generics which most stores place immediately adjacent to the branded items. You'll see that they are exactly the same. The store would rather sell the generics because they get a better margin of profit, and at the same time you may save up to 30% on the cost.

Another ploy is to talk to the pharmacist and find out if they can order some items from a generic house for you. For instance you may find that Senna-S (a stool softener) is sold pre-packed in the shelves for a crazy high price. But there are suppliers such as Goldline who also supply them in bottles of 100 tablets at a much lower price. These are usually ordered by druggists who are going to dispense them in smaller lots, but you can buy the whole bottle at a very low price.

Say you are taking something like Celexa 20mg a dose. The cost of the 40mg tabs is just a little more than for the 20's and this is generally true of all drugs Take a look at a Celexa 40mg and you'll find that the tablet has a score line so that it can be broken into 2 doses. Ask your doctor to write for the 40's then do some product modification at home and you now have twice as many doses for very little more cost.

And if you have burnt out your insurance coverage forget about buying a 30 day supply. Get hip to the economics of the pharmacy business. Most stores charge a dispensing fee plus the cost per tablet to derive a retail price. Their pricing formulae are a deep and dark secret and the retail clerk will not really know how they do it. But, when the druggist has to do nothing more than slap a label on a full container of something, the price starts to come down. Many drugs are prepacked in 100's, so get your doctor to write for 100 and you'll save a lot.

The insurance companies won't pay for more than a 30 day supply because they have you paying a co-pay which often absorbs quite a lot of the total cost. My insuror tried to tell me the reason they will only approve a 30 day supply is that they want my doctor to be able to review the need each month. If you believe that line then you probably also still believe in the Tooth Fairy. If you're taking a maintenance drug such as a hormone replacement or cholesterol lowering drug, and have been on it for a year or more, the chances you are going to quit in any one month are about the same as you getting elected to the Senate.

MEDICATIONS DOSAGE LOG - Make up a list of the medications being taken and the dosages. Pretty soon you'll be speaking like a doctor saying things such as "She takes 20mg, t.i.d." which just means she eats a 20 milligram pill or tablet three times a day. But, the reason you will need this log is that you are going to see more than one doctor and possibly some hospital staff on this journey. It will save them time, and help avoid complications if you can let them know right up front what medications are being taken. If you are computer savvy, make the list in your word processor so you can update it frequently. Make sure that when you revise the list you have a line at the bottom which says something like *Revised as of (insert date)*. Otherwise they'll all look the same in a short time.

MEDICATIONS DESCRIPTIONS - You may quickly find that with a dozen or more meds to keep track of that you will sometimes wonder what some pill which is not in it's jar actually might be. A few druggists will give you a print out that shows the design of the pill and the markings. If your druggist doesn't do this, then start making a list of the name of the pill, the description (round, tablet, capsule, oval, etc.), the color, and the markings which are stamped on or into the medication. If you need to restore some pills to their containers or to identify some you are not certain of this will save you a lot of frustration.

PATIENT'S CALENDAR - You're going to have more doctor appointments than you ever thought possible. A calendar is essential for both the patient and the care giver. Unfortunately, I haven't found a really good calendar software that's easy to use and revise. If you have WordPerfect you may try the Corel Central Calendar which I use.

I keep the short cut icon for it on my desktop so I don't have to wade through several layers to get to it. Here again make sure you put a revision date on it when you print and make a copy for each of you. List the doctor appointments, the lab visits, the appointments for other services and other appointments where both the patient and the care giver need to be involved, even if it's only in the capacity being the chauffeur for the day.

CONTACT LOG - Make a list of every medical provider you may need to have access to. This includes the oncologists, the primary care physicians, the specialists you may have used in the past or will now be seeing, your case manager at your insurance company, your doctors assistant or nurse, your pharmacies, and even your dentist. Include phone numbers as well as fax numbers, and if you can get the back office or direct line numbers for any of them keep that on the list as well. It's very important if you wind up in a hospital, need to let one doctor get in touch with another, or get a prescription called in right away.

BLOOD WORK LOG - You may also want to make a log of lab reports on blood work, and possibly the protein urine levels. When you go for labs ask the lab person for a copy of the report. Most can produce a report by machine in a few minutes while some other types such as pathology reports or urinalyses take longer. Your doctor looks for markers such as WBC which is white blood cells to see if you are at risk of infection, or red blood cells (RBC) and/or hemoglobulin (HgB) to see if you may be anemic. He'll also be looking at the platelet count (PLT) and Hematocrit (HCT) so you may find it helpful and interesting to be able to see just where you've been and how you're doing now.

DIARY - Some patients find it helpful to keep a diary or log of how they feel on a daily basis. I question how valuable this may be after you've been on the trail for a year or so, but if it makes you feel better then do it. The reason for the limited resource value is that while you may recall an adverse reaction to some drug 3 months ago, it's very likely that you're taking an array of drugs and nobody may know exactly which one cased the problem and if anything has changed in the interim the data is unreliable.

OTHER DOCUMENTS - While not in the record keeping category you should consider executing a Durable Power of Attorney for Medical care and a Living Will. Note that these are two different documents. The Power of Attorney permits your care giver to make decisions for you and give instructions for you if you are unable to communicate, but it is not a Living Will.

A Living Will comes into play when a patient is *in extremis* and has little time left. This is the document by which you instruct the hospital how to deal with you when death is imminent. You may require them to exercise every possible procedure to maintain life, or at the other hand of the scale to withhold any such procedure and DNR (do not resuscitate). It is your right to determine how you wish to be treated and these documents should be kept available as copies so that your care giver can submit them to a hospital should the need arise. Absent these written instructions the hospital and the medical team are required by law to follow certain procedures and to exercise their best judgement, which may not be in accord with your wishes. Almost any lawyer can easily draw up these forms for you. Actually his paralegal does all the work and you pay him. Your local library should have the State Statutes for your State and the forms will probably be found in there as well. Or, perhaps you can download the forms from the internet and they will probably be just as good and cost you nothing.

FINANCIAL PLANS

Financial needs can be a burden. I know. MM can destroy your credit rating as well as your skeletal integrity. The price of drugs can easily bankrupt you and many patients can add the cost of travel to distant centers of care and loss of income. It's very difficult to deal with but like any problem be it medical or economic, the earlier you start to address the problem the easier it will be to deal with it.

You can get most hospital costs taken care of by your insurance company. If you are covered by Medicare they will cover most. If you are ineligible for Medicare but qualify for Medicaid then that will cover a lot of it. But, there are still millions of us who fall between the cracks. Don't worry about the hospitals. Although their bills seem as if they were written to cover a dozen patients not just one, they will take what the insuror pays and wait for you to do what you can about the rest. Few of them are going to sue you or try to take your home away from you.

I don't know any physician who has declined to give care to a patient because the patient couldn't pay his co-payment requirements. I assume there are some out here but I hope I never meet one of them.

The pharmaceutical problem is quite something else. If you are able to pay they will accept every dollar you have until you have none left. They don't know you and don't know your problems. But, many of them do have Patient Assistance Programs through which you may be able to obtain their drugs at no cost. With one notable exception, I have found them to be humane, easy to deal with, and very accommodating. Usually you need to submit some brief financial info, have your doctor sign off that you are unable to pay and they will then ship the drugs to your doctor who will call you to come get them. Note: make sure you know when they are shipping and what; because sometimes these drugs can find their way into the doctor's goodie closet of samples. You want whoever receives the mail for your doctor to know that you know they're on the way and to call you.

The new drug card plans are of questionable value and begin to look like a Three Card Monty game. You pay $35 for a card which gets you a discount that may not be worth having to start with. And you're still dealing with an issuer who is processing through a Patient Benefits Management third-party which is also quite a profit center. If you are looking at these plans, sit down, pour a drink, relax, and try not to go crazy.

The much heralded revision in Medicare prescription coverage is certainly something of questionable value. The benefits here are akin to the weapons of mass destruction we heard so much about. Check it out and you'll find that you still pay quite a lot. You pay the premium and a $250 annual deductible, and then they pay 75% of your drug costs at fairly high retail prices, until your drug costs reach $2,250. But, then your coverage stops and you have to pay for the next $2,850 in drugs with no coverage. Coverage doesn't start again until drug expenditures reach $5,100. At that point when you've paid out $3,600 for prescription drugs plus $420 for premiums, you get coverage again. For the rest of that year, you pay $5 for every brand-name drug or 5 percent, whichever is greater. So when a drug may cost $2,000 for one prescription your cost would be $100. And after 365 days the whole thing starts over at zero.

Beginning June 2004, Medicare will provide $600 in 2004 and up to an additional $600 in 2005 to Medicare beneficiaries whose incomes are not more than 135 percent of the poverty line if they do not have certain other drug coverage. Not all drugs may be covered, and you need to inquire carefully if this may be available if you have occasional prescription coverage that gets reevaluated every month through Medicaid.

Where will this lead us? There are some of us who fear that as the new drug plans being initiated come into greater use that the pharmaceutical companies will start to curtail the Patient Assistance Plans, claiming there is no need for them as government has now bridged the gap. Another story from the Tooth Fairy. But, we shall have to wait and see.

Depending on where you live you may find local programs that can be of help. Some will even provide help with shopping, cooking and housekeeping. Check out local religious groups. You may not have to be a member nor even of that faith to be eligible. Check out the national organizations listed included in this book. Some will even help with travel expenses. There are some possibilities of getting air travel from Angel Flights when needed but start early and be flexible. If you need travel help check out the organizations which try to arrange that. The airlines themselves are generally of no help. For instance, Delta will not waive the 14-day advance purchase requirement to help get a patient to another city. Only if somebody dies will they grant a discount from the fully refundable high fares which they call a "bereavement fare" and which is a lot higher than what you would expect to pay.   You can try Priceline or others of that ilk, but the problem with them is you may wind up with departures at extremely inconvenient times and long layovers at airports which are not in the direct path you wish to travel.   I recall my wife scoring a ticket from Atlanta to Boston with a change of planes and layover at St. Louis. Duh!

If you've exhausted your financial means and your insurance coverage you may be eligible for Medicaid.   Medicaid is different in different states so there is no single answer that works for all of them except to understand some basic rules of government. First is: It doesn't have to make sense if it's a Rule.   Secondly: You can never be wrong by saying "No." Try to be armed with as much information as possible in regard to qualifying, before you file the applications.   It's a whole lot easier to slide through than to have to batter your way in. But, if you feel you are entitled and you are prepared to prove it, don't hesitate to file for an administrative review.   You will probably need some assistance on this inasmuch as the rules and standards are overly simplified for the public in their brochures,.but the actual formulae and standards are buried deep in a mess of regulations written in Government Gibberish which they aren't keen to release to we mere mortals.   On the other hand, you are entitled to this information under various Freedom of Information Acts and if you insist they will have to provide it.   Caveat: it may be better to find a brick wall and start banging your head against it. At least you'll feel better when you stop.

You may need to do some financial planning yourself or get some help from a knowledgeable lawyer or layperson who knows the ropes.   For instance, if you have a lot of credit card bills and you have some money in the stock market, you will probably be ineligible for any Medicaid help. But, if you close the brokerage accounts and pay off the credit cards and equity line so that your cash reserves are reduced, you may find yourself instantly eligible.   This is somewhat odd in one respect.   Assume you have a $25,000 equity line and you owe almost the whole sum.   You also have money in a brokerage account.   Close the account, pay off the equity line, qualify for the Medicaid and you can still go back and use the equity line when you need it.   As you dig into this morass of rules you'll find that prepaid funeral expenses are not counted as assets and that burial plots usually aren't.   You can transfer funds to these uses and may not have to actually put up money with some funeral home, but establish a trust which you can administer and thereby safeguard those funds. Similar tactics may apply to home ownership. You may want to talk to your lawyer about the ramifications of your home being in joint ownership with rights of survival (JTWROS) as opposed to a single name, or even in a trust.

ON THE ROAD AGAIN

Our life before MM was one life. Our life while we strive for remission is another life. And we will plan for life after Complete Remission (CR). We must think in these terms, for the struggle is intense, the risks are great, and the rewards may be greater.

Inasmuch as MM more often strikes people over the age of 50, it is more inclined to strike empty nesters. If the MM is advanced stage then living alone is not really a viable option. If the home consists of a couple, then one of them just got a new full time job called care giver. As discussed in the section of housekeeping changes, the home will change to accommodate the needs of the patient. Schedules will change. Food preferences will change. Sleep schedules will change. Activities will change.

If the patient is the husband, the care giving wife probably already does the cooking, laundry and shopping. It's really not a guy thing for most couples. But when the patient is the wife, the hubby has to learn quickly that cooking is more than just putting pepperoni on the pizza or nuking the chicken pot pie. Just learning the road map of the local grocery store is almost like trying to figure out the extra controls on the DVD player. I'm referring to those buttons you will never use because you really don't know what they do.

If the patient is advanced stage then hubby may have to consider his own employment. If he's employed outside the home it is going to be very difficult. If he works at home it really isn't going to be that much easier due to interruption of his days (and nights) but at least he doesn't have a supervisor watching the clock when he punches in. If he's retired, then he is about to come out of that retirement because care giving can be a big job when you do it right.

Travel can become quite a different experience. The patient won't be doing much of the driving so plan on shorter hauls, and more frequent rest stops. Your patient may be more comfortable with an extra seat cushion, a blanket, some small pillows and plenty of water and snacks in the car. You'll want to have water and snacks in the car even for short local transits. If going for a longer road trip consider an audio book. Your patient is probably going to fall asleep but maybe the book will give the driver something to get involved with.

Air travel today can be a nightmare at any time due to extensive waits for check-in and for security clearance. If your patient can't stand comfortably for prolonged times or can't walk easily for long distances, then consider telling the airline you need a porter with a wheelchair. They'll be happy to have one at your disposal and you'll go right to the head of the security clearance line because the porters want to get back to service the next customer who might just be a good tipper, too. If you have airline miles, use them to upgrade to first class because your patient is going to be a lot more comfortable than back in the cattle car. Tell the airline you will need a wheelchair at the arrival gate and they'll have one there for you, sooner or later.

If you have to rent a car make sure you rent one that's easier for your patient to get into and out of. Some of the real economy cars are designed for dwarfs and not for people with vertebral fractures and aching hips and legs. If you have a handicap parking indicia issued by your home State, be sure to take it with you when you travel. We made a color copy of ours, so we can use that on the road. You're probably not supposed to make a copy, but then you really aren't hurting anybody by doing so. If you forget it in the rental car you'll still have the original one at home.

Hotels have HC (handicapped) rooms available. Consider asking for one of these because they usually come with a much larger bathroom which will feature a walk-in shower with hand rails. The doors are larger to permit wheelchair access. Other than that, the rooms tend to be about the same as their regular rooms.

We've tried to stay at hotels which offer some sort of in-room food storage and preparation equipment. It's a big help when you can whip up a protein drink, a cup of tea, some mac and cheese or other snack, without having to order from room service. If you're staying for several nights try to get a real suites hotel with a door between the bedroom and living room. That way, if your patient needs to sleep and the care giver doesn't, he/she can read or watch TV without annoying the other person. I phrased it as "real suites" because some of the hotels which claim to be suites are not. They have a sleeping alcove without a wall and door, or some just have a kitchenette and think that makes them a suite. Embassy Suites is one chain that always has real suites. As for the others, if you don't know the property be sure to ask what the layout is.

One other thing about hotels. It's a big help if they have a breakfast buffet. Many times the patient is going to want to eat in the room and the care giver can go down and grab some chow to bring back up.   Beats having to drive to McDonald's.   Here again, what some hotels call a Continental Breakfast must be from continent called Mork, because it may be doughnuts, toast, plastic wrapped muffins, coffee and orange juice.   Not exactly the bill of fare you need for a patient, and certainly not what is offered on the Continent.

FINAL DAYS

The end may not be in sight. But, sooner or later we each reach our final days, and none of us has a contract specifying how many years, months and days we shall remain on this earth. MM patients are painfully aware of their own mortality, as are their loving care givers.

As care giver you may be loathe to discuss wishes for the final days. You know that you want to always project a positive mental attitude and help your patient be on the best emotional footing. I know that one time Phyllis and I were returning home from a long visit at an out of state hospital. We had a ten hour drive. As I entered some traffic which required my attention she started to bring up the subject of her funeral arrangements. I used the traffic as an excuse not to discuss the matter at that time, asking Little Mary Sunshine to please bag it while I paid attention to the roadway rodeo in which we found ourselves competing.

I know now that I was right and I was wrong. It is not a subject to be discussed unless the two parties can be facing or near one another and pay attention solely to the subject at hand. It is a subject that is better discussed on a good day as opposed to a day when your patient is bummed out. But, I owe a debt of gratitude to a wonderful woman who runs a local MM support group. She told me I was wrong. She told me that we should discuss it, should reduce Phyllis' desires to a written memo and then put it in the vault, or on the mantle or somewhere safe and it was over and done with and needn't be a cause of concern again. I've since spoken with other families where MM has been an uninvited guest and I know now that the advice I was given was good advice.

As a care giver you will fight the feelings of inadequacy that haunt you in your efforts to ease your patient's burden and keep your patient with you. The medical folks really won't have any definite prognosis until and unless there is nothing more that they can do, and then it is the time when you want to make the end of the journey as easy and loving as possible.

Doctors have a couple of dilemmas. Compassion vs. Law is one of them. They may feel a patient has a great chance of a seven year survival. Can they guarantee that? No they can't. Everything can change tomorrow. In most instances they will share information which they would give to the patient, with the care giver. But there could be comments they would make to a patient that they are hesitant to make to any third person.   Let your doctors know that you are a couple and that truth is what you want, be it good or not so good.

Compassion vs. Truth is a real dilemma for doctors.   If your experience with a patient in a similar circumstance suggests to you that this patient has a poor chance of an Overall Survival (OS) of more than 13 months, do you say so right up front and thereby plunge that patient into depression? Or do you dodge the issue and discuss alternative treatments and quote statistics for accepted studies?   These, as stated, are arithmetic means, and may have absolutely nothing to do with your patient who may have a vastly different expectation of Event Free Survival (EFS), or even of Quality of Life (QOL).

And because so many MM patients are parents of grown children who have their own families, you must deal with how and what to tell the kids.   Those "kids" are probably in their 40's but they're still your kids.   They deserve to know the truth and are entitled to know it. Remember that the MM experience is going to try your mental abilities to recall all the details of what you are going through, and remember that the first need of a good liar is a good memory, and then you'll see it's so much easier to tell it like it is.

I made a commitment to our children that I would never lie to them about their mother. I keep them informed of every change and the status of her health. Our daughter who lives 1,000 miles away understands that should she ever receive an email or a call that she should come to us without delay, that she should do exactly that. In return I have the comfort of knowing that all I will ever have to do is just initiate that call and her mother will have the comfort of seeing her daughter when she needs to.

Well that's it. We started this trip with the onset of a pernicious disease called Multiple Myeloma, and we've traveled a long, frightening and frustrating road to wherever it may lead. What Phyllis and I wish for each of you is that your days be filled with as much kindness and goodness as possible, that your pain be lessened, your mind be eased, and a cure for this damn disease found as soon as possible.

Please feel free to write to us with any comments and suggestions as to how to make this handbook more helpful.

GLOSSARY

It would fill a text book to list every conceivable term which you might encounter relating to MM. But, here are some more common ones and you can always ask your doctors or consult the internet sources for some of the more obscure terms.

Adhesion molecules: these allow cells to react to one another and to grow

Amyloidosis: is a disorder in which insoluble protein fibers are deposited in tissues and organs, impairing their function

Anemia: lower red blood cell count

Angiogenisis: the formation of new blood vessels, the use of drugs to thwart this is used in chemo to deny blood to new myeloma cells

Antibody: immunoglobulins made by plasma cells to help protect against infection or disease

B cell: white blood cell from which plasma cells are derived

Bence Jones Protein: a myeloma protein found in urine which serves as a marker for MM

Beta 2-microglobulin (B2M or β_2M): a protein marker used in classifying myeloma stages

Bone marrow: the soft inner core of bones, where blood cells are produced

BUN or blood urea nitrogen: a marker in the blood which may indicate kidney impairment

Calcium: higher levels indicate possible bone destruction

CAT scan: (may also be called CT scan) and is computerized axial tomography which renders 3D images of the area

CBC or complete blood count: measures various aspects of blood including white cells, red cell, platelets, hemoglobin and hematacrit as well as other indicators

Chromosome: the thing in the cell which holds the generic data

Creatinine: derived from muscles, usually filters out, elevated levels may indicate kidney trouble

CRP or C-reactive protein: a marker which indicates possible inflammations or growths in body

Electrophoresis: lab test that measures levels of various blood proteins

GEP or gene expression profile: a new approach to determining status and potential efficacy of various therapies for MM patients, based on extensive examination of the genes collected in a bone marrow biopsy

Hypercalcemia: condition caused by higher calcium levels due to bone destruction

Interleukin 6 (IL-6): a cytokine which promotes grown of MM cells

Light chain: usually called kappa or lambda light chains, are protein chains made by myeloma cells

MGUS: monoclonal gammopathy of undetermined significance, asymptomatic, with some monoclonal presence in blood or urine. Must be watched as may become full blown MM

Monoclones: identical immunoglobulins produced by MM cells and used as marker to show amount of MM in the patient

MRI or magnetic resonance image: a bone image akin to x-ray but using magnetic energy to create image

Mucositis :a complication of some cancer therapies in which the lining of the digestive system becomes inflamed or mouth sores develop

Osteoblasts: bone building cells

Osteoclasts: bone destroying cells, but work with osteoblasts to rebuild bones

Osteolytic lesion: or may be called lytic lesion, soft tumors in the bones where they have been eaten away by the MM

Plasma cell: the antibody creating immune cell derived from a B-cell

Plasmacytoma: a single tumor of malignant plasma cells, may be precursor of MM

Platelets: the stuff in blood that help it to clot

Red blood cells: the cells which carry oxygen throughout the body

Refractory: not responsive to therapies or may even be relapsed

Relapse: the return of a disease heretofore in remission, or progression of same disease

Salvage therapy: distressing name for second-line treatment for patients who did not respond well the first time around

Stem cell: the mother cell from which red, whites and platelets are created.

Stromal cell: the bone cells which help house and nourish blood producing cells

White blood cell: may be called a leukocyte and creates the immunoglobulins to fight disease

HOW TO INTERPRET YOUR CBC REPORT

In most cases the CBC is run on automated equipment and the report is generated showing the various elements of the blood which are measured as well as the accepted normal range of these elements. The elements are abbreviated, so here is the explanation of those most relevant to a MM patient.

HCT hematacrit

HGB hemoglobin

MCH means cell hemoglobin

MCHC means cell hemoglobin concentration

MCV means cell volume

MPV means platelet volume

PLT platelets

RBC red blood cell count

RDW red cell distribution width

WBC white blood cell count

126

USEFUL FORMS

At the very end of the book you will find several forms. If you enlarge these forms 150% to 155% they should work just fine on 8.5 x 11 inch paper.

The PROVIDER page just shows an imaginary list of providers and numbers which you may need to give to any other provider who needs access to some of them.   Try to include fax numbers where possible. I suggest you keep such a form in your computer but if you don't use the computer just write it out and make some copies so that when you need them for somebody you have them immediately at hand.

The PILL ROUTINES format is just an idea of what you can do in your own computer so that you will have an up to date written regimen which you can give to a physician or other medical provider.   What's importnat is the information contained in it, and not the format. Please yourself. Note that I put in an UPDATE date so that it serves to remind us to get rid of the older ones. Inasmuch as I keep in the computer I also put in the location of the file as shown lower right, so I know which one of the documents it is without having to open a bunch of them to find it.

The MED REGISTER is what we have used to track the cost of prescriptions for various vendors. I keep mine in the computer just as line entries and I alphabetize them and them insert them chronologically so that I not only can see what they cost but know when I last purchased them. If you don't want to keep the register in your computer as a document you may wish to print out the Meds Register Form which follows it, and just fill it in manually.

MEDS USAGE RECORDS may come in handy when you are on some special medication which is not a part of an ongoing regimen. Here's a form that you can easily fill in to indicate the prescription and strength and then indicate the dates when taken.

The BLOOD LABS SUMMARY is a convenient way to keep track of where you are in the blood work. It's a lot easier than leafing through a dozen pages and trying to recall what each particular was as you do so. The more important markers are arrayed to the left side of the form.

The CALENDAR form is just a universal blank calendar on which you can insert the dates and the notes for appointments and special events. Here again, the update space is very useful so you can always know if you are looking at the latest version.

If you use your browser to go to a storage site, you can directly download the forms to your computer or printer. The URL is:
www.mydocsonline.com/pub/mmforms/dwnld.pdf

ACKNOWLEDGMENTS

The learning curve for MM is steep and confusing. I'm no genius; just a guy who is making this trip with a wonderful woman and in the process of trying to understand the little bit I have managed to learn I must give sincere and grateful thanks to the people who have been of great help.

Foremost among them are two incredible ladies who head up the MM foundations. Susie Novis of the International Myeloma Foundation and Kathy Giusti of the Multiple Myeloma Research Foundation. These women are not just administrators. They know MM first hand from the experiences of their own lives and their selfless devotion to finding a cure for this disease is an inspiration to anybody who has had the honor to know them.

There have been a lot of people in the medical arena who have been of great help and support to Phyllis and me but to avoid this acknowledgment becoming an unsolicited testimonial I refer to them obliquely because they will know who they are, while leaving you the choice of providers.

Dr. B and Bonnie for their loving attention even though their schedules are such that they could work 80 hour weeks and still not find the top of their desks.

Dr. F and Rhonda for their constant attention to every little problem as well as the big ones. Rhonda is the kind of special RN who always anticipates what the doctor wants and has it done before he can ask for it.

Mary Anne Valdecanas for being the absolutely brilliant physician who first found the M spike and got us on the road before any more damage could occur.

To Ted Goff who graciously allowed the use of his cartoon on the front cover so that we could inject a bit of humor into this grim situation. Thank you, Ted.

And to the nice folks at mydocsonline.com. They electronically store documentation for their corporate clients and are storing our forms so you can print them out whenever you need them.

And to the many friends and family members who had stood by our side for more than a year and given their support in the form of chicken soup, visits, cards, financial help and so much more.

We thank you all.

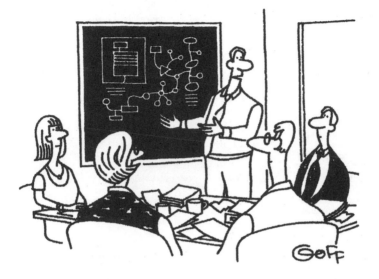

There! Now that I've
laid it all out for you,
it's a lot easier to
understand. Right?

Meds list for   Updated to June 11, 2004
Patricia Patient

Maintainance Meds   (all i.i.d unless noted)

Caltrate	600+D
Multivitamin	see attached profile sheet
Maxide	25 mg
Prevacid	30 mg
Armour thyroid	120 mg
Prometrium	100 mg
Cenestin	625 mg
Celexa	20 mg

Temporary Meds   *(Italics = not currently used much)*

Duragesic patch	50 mcg	replace every third day
Dexamethasone	40 mg	cycles days 1-4, 9-12 of 28 day cycle
Thalidomide	100 mg	i.i.d.
Warfarin	1 mg	i.i.d.
Miralax	17mg	q.i d
Lorazapam	*1 mg*	*as needed for nausea*

Doctors

PCP	Susan Graceland	404-515-8944	
	Fax	404-988-6551	
Hema/Oncol	Bernie Softwords	404-471-5213	Nurse is x 5, 2
	Nurse Sophie's FAX	404-987-6541	
Radio/Oncol	Laser Blazer	678-123-4567	
	Blazer - cell phone	432-456-7890	
GYN	Mary Feelgood	988-854-7412	
Neuro Surgeon	Paul Stickem	404-255-5511	
	Stickem - Fax	404-255-1155	
Dermatology	Dontcha Pickett	770-554-4455	
Surgeon	Lace Allott	404-444-4114	
Pain Management	Ike M. Easem	404-963-2587	Erma is X 505

Druggist	Publix	770-123-4567
	Publix Rx fax	770-987-6543
	Costco	770-352-8677

Insurance	Blue Cross / Blue Shield of xxx	800-444-5555
	Member Nbr 14589756-887	
	Group Nbr 888GP-4	
	Case Manager - Cheryl Raven	800-588-7895 x4517
	Fax	404-777-9995

PILL ROUTINES (UPDATED AS OF July 9, 2004)

Daily in Morning:
Caltrate
Vitamin
Maxide   25
Prevacid   30
Thyroid
Celexa   40
Coumadin   1

Daily mid-day:

Daily at night:
Prometrium   100
Cenestin   0.625
Xanax   1

Take as Needed:
Carafate (1 hour before meals)   q.i.d.   1gm
Ativan   p.r.n.   1mg
Xanax   p.r.n.   0.25 mg
Duagesic (every 3 days)   25/50 mcg
Senna
Senna-S
Stool softener

SPECIAL NOTES:

Dex (5 tabs) Days 1-4, 9-12 of each 28 day cycle

MEDS REGISTER

Rx		QTY	VENDOR	PRICE	DATE
alprazolam (XANAX)	1 mg	30	Publix	4.94	6/14
armour thyroid	120 mg	30	Publix	8.76	8/02
armour thyroid	120 mg	30	Publix	8.76	8/26
celexa	20 mh	30	Publix	64.43	8/13
cenestin	0.625 mg	30	Publix	23.07	7/19
cenestin	0.625	15	Publix	12.16	9/16
dexamethasone	4 mg	120	Publix	21.33	7/19
difulucan	100/50	2	Publix	16.46	8/23
difulucan	100/50	2 each	2	Publix	24.07	9/16
duragesic	50 McG	5	Publix	105.08	6/13
duragesic	25 McG	5	Publix	62.35	6/30
hydrocodone	10-650	30	Publix	14.95	7/18
hydrocodone	10-500	30	Kmart	14.29	5/20
lactulose	1 liter	1	Costco	34.49	6/30
levaquin	500 mg	7	Publix	60.50	7/11
lorazepam (ativan)	1mg	12	CVS	3.73	9/12
lorazepam (ativan)	1mg	30	Publix	6.08	10/05
lorazepam (ativan)	1mg	100	Publix	13.28	10/22
maxide (generic)	37.5-5.25	45	Publix	10.02	8/23
miralax	powder	255 gm	Publix	19.50	10/31
mycelex	10 mg	10	Publix	15.42	8/20
Mycelex	10 mg	100	Costco	163.42	8/20

MEDS REGISTER

Rx	Strength	Qty	Vendor	Price	Date

This page

intentionally

left blank

MEDICATION USAGE RECORD for _____

MEDICATION	DATE	DATE	DATE	DATE	DATE	DATE	DATE	DATE

Notes:

This page

intentionally

left blank

Blood Labs Summary

DATE	WBC	RBC	HCT	PLT	HGB	MPV	MCV	MCH	MCHC	RDW

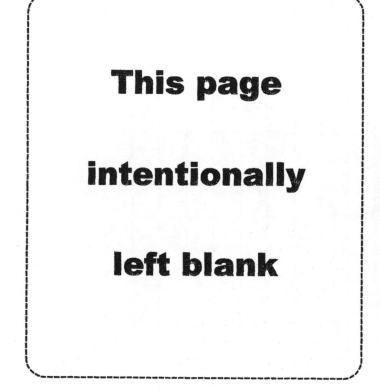

This page

intentionally

left blank

Calendar

Edited through _____

SUNDAY	MONDAY	TUESDAY	WEDNESDAY	THURSDAY	FRIDAY	SATURDAY

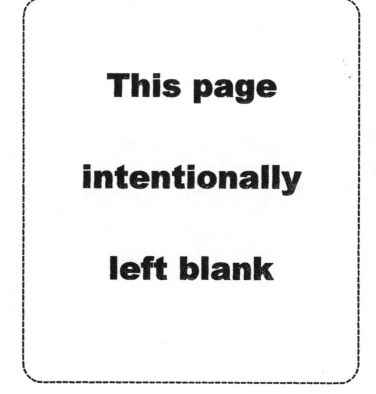

This page

intentionally

left blank

STOP PRESS !

As we go to press we have cause to have great concern about a condition which may plague many MM patients. It is **xerostomia**, or more commonly referred to as dry mouth.

Few of the doctors caring for MM patients will ever bother to carefully inspect your dentures or specifically warn you about the dangers of dry mouth as a result of the disease progression, radiation, or some of the medications being introduced into your system.

Dry mouth is **NOT** like nausea or fatigue which may go away with time after the medication is discontinued. It is a dangerous risk of permanent dental destruction and you need to be aware of it.

None of those little yellow stickers on the prescription bottles will raise a warning for this problem. Some of the print-outs that come with the medication may list dry mouth as a possible side effect. Dry mouth doesn't seem to raise any alarm bells but it should.

Thalidomide is now back as an approved medication but it is supplied with very carefully packed warnings because of the terrible dangers which can accompany it.

Not unlike the fetal birth defects which were caused by thalidomide, xerostomia is a PERMANENT disability that will not just go away and may involve you in thousands of dollars of reconstruction work and throw you into fits of despair and anxiety. Of course, some of those anxiety meds can contribute to xerostomia so this is a real Catch-22.

The problem is compounded by lack of public data. The Physician Prescribing Information format dictated by the FDA only requires that side effects be reported in categories, such as having affected more than 10% of patients in the clinical trial group. Of course, that could be 11% or 99% and finding out the actual percentages isn't an easy job.

Further aggravation is attributable to the insurors, whether they be private plans or Medicare, which do not cover restorative dental work. Regardless that the damage is directly attributable to the disease or therapy and not to your negligence, most will turn you away without consideration.

Best advice is to make sure you get complete and careful dental assessment quite often. Perhaps as often as 4 times a year; because the damage from xerostomia may occur as much as a year after starting to use some of these meds, and can manifest itself in as little as a 3 month period.

If you are a MM patient and think you have suffered serious dental destruction due to medications, or want more info you may want to check the website **drymouth.org** for more information.

NOTES

NOTES

NOTES

NOTES

NOTES